GAPS INTRODUCTION DIET COOKBOOK

100 Delicious & Nourishing Recipes for Stages 1 to 6

Andre Parker

RECOMMENDED AND CERTIFIED BY THE EXPERTS

It's a joy to see a cookbook that is so well laid out, so easy to follow. Andre has worked hard to make this work GAPS compliant. What a pleasure it is to see a GAPS cookbook which is so thorough and complete. The only difficult thing was reading through but wanting to continually stop to go cook some of the delicious looking recipes. When doing GAPS, it's often difficult because you can't think. This is a great book to assist in those troubling days.

Becky Plotner
ND, tdnl nat, CGP, D.PSc
https://www.nourishingplot.com/

TABLE OF CONTENTS

PRAISE FOR GAPS INTRODUCTION DIET COOKBOOK

I am a huge fan of Andre's. When you begin on the GAPS diet is can be so overwhelming and Andre's cookbooks just simplify the whole process. He really is a life saver and I always recommend his books to my clients (I'm a Nutritionist). Recipes are simple and easy to follow which is always a blessing when beginning a new way of eating. Thank you for another amazing book Andre!!!

Miss W.
Amazon Customer Review

This little GAPS cookbook has breathed new life into my "intro" repertoire. I'm eating the chicken-cauli tabbouleh tonight and it is wonderful. I have multiple pages bookmarked to try. This book has given me the encouragement I need to carry on and stick to the GAPS diet. Thanks, Andre!

Heather Lasher
Amazon Customer Review

The Gaps Diet, has helped so many people heal from chronic digestive problems, as well as various mental/emotional problems. The main book written on Gaps is fantastic but a bit daunting. It is long, in depth, and can be a bit overwhelming to figure out where to begin. This book makes it SO simple. Its easily breaks down how Gaps intro stage, and filled with easy to make recipes. Having one 100 recipes helps to remove the restrictive feelings that may come with starting the diet, and helps to remove much of the overwhelm. I recommend not only for beginners but for experienced Gap dieters as well, for the recipes.

Emily
Amazon Customer Review

I'm overjoyed that Andre took the time to write this book. This easy to read and understand book is turning my overwhelmingly, confusing and complicated GAPS journey into a well-organized, simplified one!! WHAT A RELIEF!

Thank you Andre.

Terreca Marlene Stuck
Amazon Customer Review

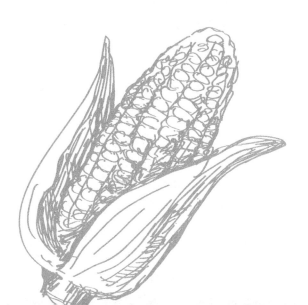

THANK YOU

I want to thank you for purchasing this book and I really hope it helps you keep to your health goals. The GAPS diet completely turned my life around and I am now healthy and fit thanks to this diet. I have been compelled to write this book by my desire to help others benefit from the GAPS diet in the life-changing way that it has helped me. I hope that these easy but delicious recipes will inspire you to start or continue with the GAPS diet and put you on the road to a healthier, more active and more fulfilling life.

I would love to hear about your story and how the GAPS diet has helped you or a loved one so please feel free to email me at the address below.

If you enjoyed this book or have any suggestions, I would be very grateful if you would leave a review or simply e-mail me your feedback.

You can leave a review on Amazon at the link below:
https://andreparker.co/gapsintroreview

Or email me at:
info@andreparker.co

Warmest Regards,
Andre

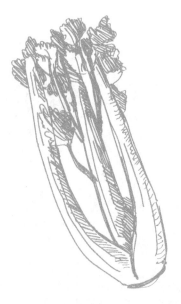

INTRODUCTION

I wanted to write this cookbook for every single one of you embarking on the introduction stage of the diet, whether it is for the very first time or a re-run through the most challenging – but also the most essential – part of the GAPS diet.

Having gone through the GAPS introduction diet, as well as the Full GAPS diet, I know how hard it is to get through the introduction stages, both physically AND mentally.

The introduction stages are designed to repair all of the damage that has been wreaked on your gut for years and the repair process is a tough one!

To this date, getting through the GAPS diet and repairing my (much damaged) gut remains one of the hardest physical and mental things that I have ever done in my entire life.

I would like to take this opportunity to say that I have a deep level of respect and admiration for you for embarking on this journey. It will be a tough journey, but I sincerely hope I can assist you in your journey by offering delicious and nutritious GAPS-compliant recipes!

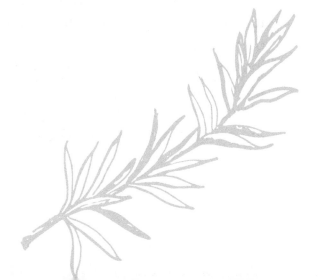

WHAT IS THE GAPS DIET?

Many of you have probably already heard of the GAPS diet, but you may still be wondering exactly what this diet is all about. You may know that this diet was created as a way to restore gut health - but there is a lot more to it than that. If the GAPS diet is somewhat confusing or brand new to you, don't worry. I am going to get down to the basics and really break down what this diet is all about. Diets can be confusing but I promise you won't be confused by the end of section.

GAPS stands for Gut and Psychology Syndrome and it was developed by Dr. Natasha Campbell-McBride MD. The GAPS diet was derived from the SCD (Specific Carbohydrate Diet) as a way of naturally treating inflammatory diseases, such as those in the digestive tract. Dr. Campbell-McBride took the SCD diet and adjusted it to fit the healthcare needs of her patients who were suffering from a combination of various digestive and neurological conditions that resulted from an imbalance in the bacterial ecosystem that lives in the gastrointestinal tract. The new protocol that Dr. Campbell-McBride would go on to call the GAPS diet. An interesting fact about the name of this diet is that Dr. Campbell-McBride didn't call it the GAPS diet originally. It was a name her patients called it which she coined as the official name after a couple of years. The GAPS diet focuses on removing foods from the diet that are very difficult to digest, as well as foods that are known to cause damage to the gut flora in your digestive tract. The GAPS diet focuses on replacing these gut-depriving and damaging foods with foods that are not only incredibly nutrient-dense but foods that will also allow the intestinal lining of the gut a chance to heal. With Intestinal Permeability on the rise, it's never been more important to find a diet that is going to focus on healing the gut and on foods that are going to give the digestive system the boost that it needs to thrive.

Since this diet has such as specific approach to helping neurological as well as digestive conditions, there are very specific foods that are off limits in the GAPS diet. There are also various stages of this diet, where GAPS-compliant foods are gradually introduced into the diet.

It is important to emphasize at this point that, no matter what stage of the diet you are in, steering clear of processed foods is essential. There are far too many convenient food options in today's society and the majority of these are highly processed. Processing food changes both its chemical and its biological structure, and it also depletes the food of the nutritional value it once had. It's also important not to forget that our bodies were not designed to digest processed foods that have been changed and tampered with from their original state.

On top of this, chemicals are added to processed foods in order to add in flavors and colors that have been lost due to processing. These chemicals have been shown to cause hyperactivity and learning disabilities, among various other health conditions. Our digestive system also takes a massive hit when we consume processed and chemical-laden foods. No matter what stage of the GAPS diet you are in, processed foods must be eliminated in order to heal.

Sugar is another food that must be eliminated from your diet. Not only is sugar incredibly addictive, but sugar has a very adverse effect on gut flora, which can be even worse for anyone who already suffers from digestive issues. Soya is unfortunately another major problem and should be avoided altogether. Most of the food manufacturing industry unfortunately uses genetically modified soya and it is also very high in phytates, which are substances that are naturally found in the bran of all grains. The issue with phytates is that they can bind to minerals and then prevent them from being absorbed. Many people following the GAPS diet may already be deficient in certain vitamins and minerals, so a food that is going to strip your body of the vitamins and minerals that it needs to thrive should be completely bypassed.

Wheat will also need to be removed from your diet when following the GAPS protocol. Gluten-free diets have been shown to improve symptoms associated with certain conditions such as autism and even schizophrenia, as well as digestive issues. Refined gluten containing carbohydrates such as white bread, white pasta and other refined products feed parasites as well as harmful bacteria, not to mention the issues it can cause with candida overgrowth. For this reason, gluten and wheat products are kept out of the GAPS diet to prevent further damage to an already sensitive and potentially toxin-ridden body. Wheat is also a very common food allergy and sensitivity, so it is best to avoid it in any event, especially during the healing process.

I hope that you are starting to get excited about the GAPS diet. This diet completely changed my life and I am hopeful that it will do the same for you!

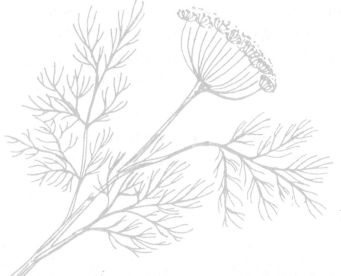

THE GAPS INTRODUCTION DIET

Each stage of the GAPS diet allows for a gradual re-introduction of different foods. Therefore, Stage 1 of the GAPS diet is the stage where you are most restricted and you will likely find it to be the most challenging. The sudden change in coming off a diet that was probably loaded with foods that did not sit well with your body can be tough and may lead to some detox symptoms where you feel intense cravings at times. The grass is truly greener on the other side, so please stick with it. The introduction diet, if done right, will keep you very well nourished and hydrated, which is exactly what your body needs during the adjustment period. To set yourself up for success, it is a good idea to prep a couple of homemade stocks ahead of time and to be prepared with lots of GAPS- approved vegetables before you get started. This way, you can grab and go, and it doesn't take ages to put your meals together. Stage 1 is a very basic diet and consists of the following foods:

Introduction Diet: Stage 1

- Homemade meat stock
- Meats & fish cooked into the stock such as:
  - Beef
  - Lamb
  - Chicken
  - Turkey
  - Fish

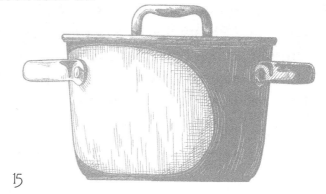

15

- Non-fibrous vegetables cooked in the stock, these can include:
  - Collard greens
  - Bok choy
  - Kale
  - Spinach
  - Zucchini
  - Pumpkin
  - Summer squash
  - Onion
  - Garlic
  - Carrots
  - Broccoli
  - Cauliflower
  - Fermented vegetable juice
  - Turnips

Please note that if you're suffering from extreme cases of diarrhea, it is recommended that you exclude vegetables at first and focus on stock with probiotic-rich foods every hour with well-cooked meats and fish. You will not want to introduce vegetables until after the diarrhea begins to calm down. You want to reduce that inflammation before adding in the fiber.

Fermented yogurt & dairy – Only include a small amount each day. Some people do ok starting with a drop while others start with a teaspoon. However, keep in mind that there are many people who are not able to progress this quickly, so progress as your body allows. Homemade is best, and you can find a homemade recipe in the recipe section of this book. You may also want to consider adding in some whey, sour cream, or kefir. It's important to remember that only fermented dairy is GAPS approved, and that things like raw dairy would be something to consider adding only after you are coming off of the GAPS diet. Again, quality is key here, so you will want to opt for the highest quality possible. This may be a great option for those who suffer from diarrhea.

Other fermented foods - there are other ways to get probiotic-rich foods into your diet. The juice from your homemade sauerkraut or fermented vegetables is an excellent option. Try adding these to your soup for an extra probiotic-rich boost. These are the best fermented options if you suffer from constipation.

Ginger, mint or chamomile tea - you can sweeten your tea with a small amount of raw and local honey if desired. Be sure to use the whole leaf version of tea and not the powdered version.

The GAPS introduction diet focuses on nourishing foods that nourish the gut lining with things like amino acids, fats, vitamins, and minerals. The foods help to renew the gut lining. The introduction part of the GAPS diet also initially removes any fiber, as well as other substances that may cause irritation to the gut and could ultimately interfere with the healing process. Not everyone knows that they have inflammation in the gut so, by focusing on the nourishing and supporting foods, the gut is allowed to heal even in cases where inflammation has gone undetected. The GAPS introduction diet also includes probiotic-rich, healthy bacteria right from the get-go so the gut can start repairing itself and heal with beneficial bacteria.

Once the introduction phase of this diet begins, you can decide to move through the diet as fast as your body permits. You may wish to stay at different stages for different periods of time. Listen to your body and move through at the pace you feel is best. The most important thing to remember is to take the introduction diet seriously and not to skip it or rush through it. The introduction phase of the GAPS diet is integral to success and, by following this part of the diet, you allow your digestive system to begin the healing process quicker than you would if you completely skipped over it. Stick to each stage of the introduction diet for at least a few days to help improve symptoms before moving to the next stage.

Stage 2:

Now that you have made it to Stage 2, you are probably hoping that you can add a bit more into your diet! If you've made it to this stage, you are also probably starting to feel better and you are probably starting to get excited about the amazing possibilities this diet has to heal your gut. If you've had some detoxifying symptoms or "die-off", this is great as well because it is a sign that your body is getting rid of the toxins and getting better. For Stage 2, you will still want to be enjoying your soups boiled with meats, vegetables and probiotic-rich foods. You will probably want to gradually add some raw pasture raised organic eggs into the soups at this point. It's important to only add the egg yolks into the soups, removing the egg whites. You can start with one egg yolk per day and then gradually increase it until you are enjoying an egg for each bowl of soup you enjoy. Stick with organic, pasture-raised eggs. At this stage, you can also add in some stews and casseroles made with meats and vegetables but avoid any spices in Stage 2. You will also want to continue to increase the amount of homemade whey, sour cream, yogurt or kefir in your diet as well as the juice from your homemade sauerkraut and fermented vegetables. You can also add in one small piece of fermented fish per day in Stage 2 such as Swedish gravlax. Homemade ghee can be introduced here at one teaspoon per day and then gradually increased.

Stage 3:

Welcome to Stage 3! You have started adding more foods into your diet, as you steadily increase the amount of probiotic-rich foods in your diet as well. On Stage 3, you will want to continue with the foods you have been eating and you can now add a ripe avocado mashed into your soups and egg whites after egg yolks are tolerated. Start with about 1–3 teaspoons per day. You can now even make GAPS-approved pancakes at this stage, made from nut butter, eggs and summer squash like zucchini! You can find a recipe in the recipes section to get started. You may also start making scrambled eggs, cooked in ghee or pork fat, and served with avocado and even some cooked onion. Lastly, start to actually eat the fermented vegetables and sauerkraut instead of only enjoying the juice. Start small and work your way up to having 1–4 teaspoons at each meal.

Stage 4:

At Stage 4, you will want to gradually increase cooked meats by roasting and grilling them instead of only cooking them in your soups. However, keep in mind that grilling in the GAPS diet refers to grilling in the UK which involves food put in the oven with heat coming down on the food from the top, as in cooking in an oven. Enjoy cooked meats with cooked vegetables as well as sauerkraut. You can now also begin enjoying freshly-pressed juice by starting with a very small amount of carrot juice. Once you are comfortable having a full cup of fresh carrot juice per day, you can branch out and try celery, cabbage, lettuce and mint juices as well. At Stage 4 you are also welcome to add in cold- pressed olive oil, working your way up to 1–2 tablespoons for each meal. Lastly, you can start to bake with ground almonds by making almond bread or make the bread with any other nuts and seeds ground into flour.

Stage 5:

On Stage 5 of the GAPS diet, you will want to continue to enjoy all of the nourishing foods you have already added into your diet and you can begin to add cooked apple puree. Keep an eye out for a recipe in the recipes section! You may also begin adding raw vegetables, starting with the softer parts of lettuce and cucumber. Increase the raw vegetable intake until well tolerated and, if diarrhea comes back, you know your body is not quite ready to introduce these foods yet. If the vegetable juices have been well tolerated, you can now begin to add fruits such as pineapple and mango, and other citrus fruits.

Stage 6:

You have almost completed the GAPS introduction diet! I hope that you are feeling much better and are ready to start the Full GAPS diet. On Stage 6, if all of the other foods have been well tolerated, you can now try some peeled raw apple and slowly introduce raw fruits, with a little bit more honey in your diet as well. You can also introduce baked goodies that are GAPS approved, which you will find in the recipe section of this book. For baked goods, you will want to stick to dried fruit as the sweetener.

While it may seem like six stages are quite a lot to get through, I hope that breaking down each stage makes things a little clearer. As you can see, each stage builds the stage before it and goes at a gradual pace so as not to trigger any inflammation in your body. As you progress through the diet, remember to keep enjoying the foods from the previous stage as well so you are gradually increasing the variety of food that you are eating. Listen to your body and go at a pace that works for you. Once you have finished all six stages, you are ready for the Full GAPS diet, which you will find a breeze by comparison!

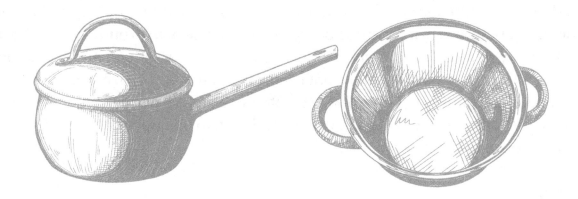

THE FULL GAPS DIET

Since this book deals with the GAPS introduction diet only, this is only intended to be a brief word on the Full GAPS diet, which you will start to follow once you have successfully completed the introductory stages.

Once you start this phase of this diet, you will be very experienced with the GAPS way of eating, and you will probably be feeling a great deal better! You will also have gained some insight as to how your body responds to certain foods. Keeping a food diary can be very helpful, especially during the introduction diet, so that you can reference back to this when you start the Full GAPS diet. This will help you pinpoint which foods agree with you and which do not.

The Full GAPS diet, once started, will need to be followed for about two years. While two years is recommended, some may stay on the diet more than two years and some for less. Some people who may have milder conditions may be able to start introducing non-allowed foods after two years on Full GAPS with no symptoms, while others will have to strictly stick to the diet for much longer. It all depends on your individual case. The general rule of thumb is to stick to the GAPS diet in its entirety for two years on Full GAPS, two years after the intro diet is completed before you start adding in non-GAPS approved foods.

A typical Full GAPS diet would look something like this: You would start your day with a glass of filtered water with either a slice of lemon or a teaspoon of apple cider vinegar. You can then enjoy a glass of fresh pressed fruit or vegetable juice. For breakfast, you can choose eggs with sausage and vegetables and some onions or even a GAPS-approved homemade muffin. For lunch, a homemade soup with some probiotic-rich foods would be great and, lastly, dinner could include a homemade stew or any meat or fish cooked with vegetables.

When you are ready to start coming off the GAPS diet, keep in mind that getting off the GAPS diet could lead to unwanted reactions if done suddenly and you need to have 2 years of normal digestion before you should even consider adding in non-GAPS foods. Sticking to the GAPS diet will also prevent you from consuming a modern diet packed with sugar and processed foods again, which is not a bad thing! Your body will become accustomed to eating the foods it's meant to, which is why adding processed junk back into your diet again could potentially cause you to feel quite ill. Keep in mind that starting the GAPS diet is incredibly rewarding for your overall health and one of the best decisions you can make for your gut health!

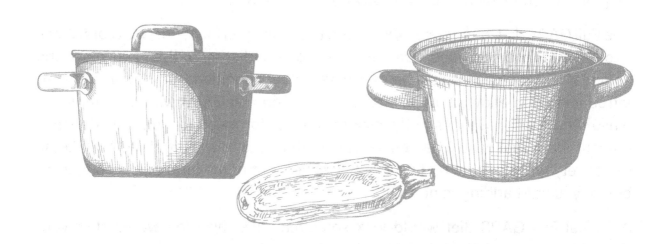

GLOSSARY OF TERMS

Grass-fed This applies to **beef, lamb and dairy products** such as milk, yogurt and cheese. It means that the cows and lambs have been allowed to graze in pasture year-round, rather than being fed a processed diet with little nutritional value for much of their life.

Organic This applies to **meat, dairy products, vegetables and fruit**. Ideally, all of the vegetables and fruit you consume should be organic but we have not specified this in the recipes. Animal products are not as important as Dr. Natasha states that because animals have their own detoxification systems, they are able to detox toxins which doesn't make purchasing organic meat as important as organic fruits and vegetables. If you have to choose between what you buy organic, meat and eggs are not as important.

Pastureraised This applies to chicken, **pork, and eggs** and means that the chickens have been free to roam on rotated pastures where they can enjoy a healthier, more natural diet of wild grasses and eggs, rather than kept in cages and fed a limited diet of corn.

Raw This is used for **milk or cream** and means that it is unpasteurized and unprocessed and therefore is richer in nutrients.

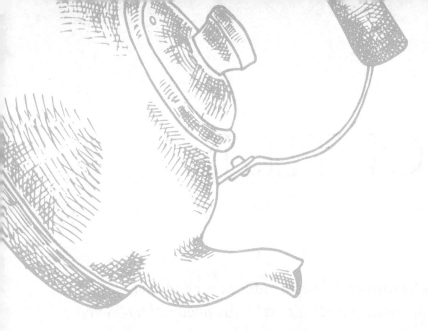

Base Recipes

GAPS CHICKEN STOCK

Serves: 8

Prep Time: 10 minutes

Cook Time: 2 hours

Tips:

- Use the meat from the chicken for some of the recipes below, such as the Chicken Carrot Soup.
- Strip off the soft tissues from the bones to later use in soups.

Ingredients:

- 1 whole organic pasture-raised chicken
- 3 carrots, chopped
- 9 cloves of garlic, chopped
- 3 sprigs of fresh rosemary
- 7 sprigs of fresh thyme
- 7 sprigs of fresh parsley
- 2 bay leaves
- 1 Tbsp. mineral salt
- Crushed peppercorn (in a cache to be easily removed)
- Filtered water

Directions:

1. Simply add the chicken to the base of a large pot and fill it with water. Add enough water to cover the chicken.

2. Add the salt, cover, and bring to a boil. Scoop off the foam on the top and then cover and simmer for two hours.

3. Once cooked, remove the chicken and peppercorn, and strain the stock.

4. Store the stock in mason jars in the refrigerator or freezer.

25

GAPS BEEF STOCK

Serves: 8

Prep Time: 10 minutes

Cook Time: 3 hours

Tips:

- Use the meat in any of the vegetable soup recipes below.
- Store the stock in the refrigerator for up to 7 days or in the freezer for a few months.

Ingredients:

- 6 organic grass-fed beef soup bones (The bones should be a mixture of joint bones, marrow bones and bones with a little bit of meat on them. The meat should be no further than an inch from the bone)
- 1 tsp. apple cider vinegar
- 1 Tbsp. mineral salt
- 1 tsp. crushed peppercorn (in a cache to be easily removed)
- Filtered water

Directions:

1. Simply add the beef soup bones to the base of a large stock pot and fill with water. Add enough water to cover the beef bones.

2. Add the salt and the apple cider vinegar. Place the stock pot over high heat but turn the heat down to low as soon as the stock starts to boil.

3. Scoop the foam off before turning it down. Simmer covered with a lid.

4. Keep it at a low simmer for about 3 hours.

5. Once the stock is cooked, strain it and divide it between mason jars.

6. Store the mason jars in the refrigerator or freezer.

FISH STOCK

Serves: 10

Prep Time: 10 minutes

Cook Time: 30-60 minutes

Ingredients:

- 2 lb. of fish fins, bones and head
- 2 carrots, chopped
- ½ bulb fennel, chopped
- 3 cloves garlic, chopped
- 2 sprigs fresh thyme
- 2 sprigs fresh parsley
- 1 bay leaf
- 1 tsp. mineral salt
- 1 tsp. crushed peppercorn (in a cache to be easily removed)

Directions:

1. Simply add all of the ingredients, except the garlic, to a large stockpot and cover with enough filtered water to cover the fish bones. Bring to a boil. Scoop the foam off, then turn down to a low simmer and put the lid on and cook for 30 minutes or an hour if using a larger fish.

2. Add the chopped garlic, bring to the boil and then turn off the heat.

3. Remove the fish fins, bones and head and strain the stock before using.

4. Freeze or refrigerate any leftover stock to have on hand when you need homemade stock and are short on time.

SAUERKRAUT JUICE

Serves: 18

Prep Time: 10 minutes + fermentation time

Cook Time: 0 minutes

Tips:

- If you want to enjoy sauerkraut juice sooner than 7–14 days, you can use a starter culture in place of the salt. If using a high-quality starter culture, you will be able to enjoy your sauerkraut within 5 days as opposed to up to two weeks.

- Make sure that soups and stews are not too hot when adding sauerkraut juice (or other probiotic foods) as the heat could destroy the beneficial probiotic bacteria.

Ingredients:

- 1 head of cabbage
- 6 Tbsp. mineral salt
- Filtered water

Directions:

1. Start by chopping the head of cabbage in a food processor or high-speed blender. You will want to cut the cabbage into smaller pieces before blending.

2. Transfer the chopped cabbage into a large mixing bowl and sprinkle with the salt. Allow this to sit for one hour.

3. Take a couple of large mason jars, fill them ⅓ of the way full with the salted cabbage and then fill the rest with the filtered water, leaving a little room at the top.

4. Cover the jars and allow them to sit for 7–14 days on the countertop.

5. After the fermentation process, store in the refrigerator and use the juice from stage 1 of the GAPS diet. The sauerkraut itself can be enjoyed from stage 3 onwards.

Stage 1

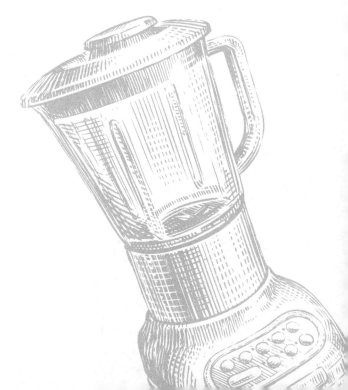

BREAKFAST

CARROT SUMMER SQUASH BREAKFAST SOUP

Serves: 2

Prep time: 15 minutes

Cook time: 20-25 minutes

Ingredients:

- 4 cups homemade stock
- 1 cup carrots, chopped
- 1 cup of summer yellow squash, peeled and cubed
- 1 clove garlic, chopped

Directions:

1. Add the stock, carrots and squash to a large stock pot and bring to a boil.

2. Reduce to a simmer and cook for 20-25 minutes or until the vegetables are tender.

3. Add the chopped garlic, bring to the boil and then turn off the heat.

4. Using an immersion blender, blend until smooth.

GINGER AND CHAMOMILE TEA

Serves: 1

Prep time: 5 minutes

Cook time: 0 minutes

Ingredients:

- 1 tsp. fresh ginger, grated
- 1 sachet fresh loose leaf chamomile tea
- 1 tsp. raw honey

Directions:

1. Bring a pot of water to a boil and add the grated ginger and chamomile tea to a mug.

2. Add the boiling water to the mug and steep for 3-5 minutes.

3. Remove the chamomile leaf sachet and pour the tea through a sieve.

4. Sweeten with the raw honey and enjoy.

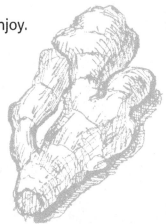

BREAKFAST YOGURT

Serves: 8

Prep time: 15 minutes + fermentation time (24 hours +)

Cook time: 10 minutes

Tips:

- Where possible, use raw organic milk as this is much richer in nutrients since it has not been pasteurized or processed. However, raw milk does not get heated prior to the starter. More starter is needed with raw milk.

Ingredients:

- ½ gallon organic grass-fed milk
- ½ cup organic grass-fed unsweetened yogurt
- Raw honey for serving

Directions:

1. Start by heating the milk in a large stockpot, bring to a simmer at 180 degrees and then remove from the heat. Allow the milk to cool to room temperature.

2. Once cool, pour 1 cup of the milk into a mixing bowl with the half cup of yogurt.

3. Add the mixture to the stockpot with the rest of the milk and stir to combine.

4. Divide into mason jars.

5. Place the yogurt into the oven with the oven lights on but do not turn the oven on.

6. Allow the yogurt to sit in the oven for at least 24 hours and then place in the refrigerator to set.

7. Once set, enjoy with a drizzle of honey.

LUNCH

BROCCOLI SOUP

Serves: 4

Prep time: 15 minutes

Cook time: 15-20 minutes

Ingredients:

- 4 cups homemade stock
- 1 cup broccoli florets
- ½ yellow onion, chopped
- 1 clove garlic, chopped
- Sauerkraut juice as tolerated

Directions:

1. Start by adding the broccoli and onion with the meat stock to a large stock pot and bring to a boil.

2. Reduce to a simmer and cook for 15-20 minutes or until the broccoli and the chopped onion is tender.

3. Add the chopped garlic, bring to a boil again and then turn off the heat.

4. Using an immersion blender, blend until smooth and then serve with as much sauerkraut juice as tolerated. Some people start with a drop while others do ok with a teaspoon.

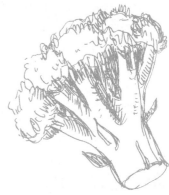

CHICKEN CARROT SOUP

Serves: 4

Prep time: 15 minutes

Cook time: 20-25 minutes

Tip:
- Use the chicken removed from the bones after making your homemade stock, if possible.

Ingredients:

- 4 cups homemade stock
- 1 cup organic pasture-raised chicken, cooked and shredded
- 1 cup carrots, chopped
- ½ yellow onion, chopped
- 1 clove garlic, chopped
- Sauerkraut juice as tolerated

Directions:

1. Start by adding the chicken, carrot and onion with the meat stock to a large stock pot and bring to a boil.

2. Reduce to a simmer and cook for 20-25 minutes or until the carrots and the chopped onion are tender.

3. Add the chopped garlic, bring to a boil again and then turn off the heat.

4. Serve with as much sauerkraut juice as tolerated. Some people start with a drop while others do ok with a teaspoon.

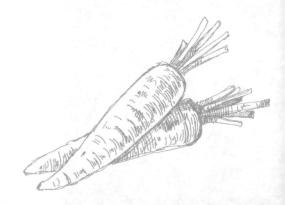

34

CAULIFLOWER SOUP

Serves: 2

Prep time: 15 minutes

Cook time: 15-20 minutes

Ingredients:

- 4 cups homemade stock
- 2 cups cauliflower florets
- ½ yellow onion, chopped
- 1 clove garlic, chopped
- Sauerkraut juice

Directions:

1. Start by adding the cauliflower and onion to a large stock pot with the meat stock and bring to a boil.

2. Reduce to a simmer and cook for 15-20 minutes or until the cauliflower and the chopped onion is tender.

3. Add the chopped garlic, bring to a boil again and then turn off the heat.

4. Using an immersion blender and blend until smooth.

5. Serve with as much sauerkraut juice as tolerated. Some people start with a drop while others do ok with a teaspoon.

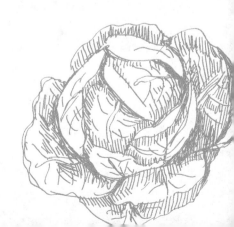

PUMPKIN SOUP

Ingredients:

Serves: 3-4

Prep time: 15 minutes

Cook time: 30 minutes

- 5 cups homemade stock
- 1 pumpkin, peeled, seeded, and chopped
- ½ yellow onion, chopped
- ½ tsp. mineral salt
- 2 cloves garlic, chopped
- Sauerkraut juice as tolerated

Directions:

1. In a large stock pot over high heat, add the stock, butternut squash, onion and salt. Bring to a boil, then reduce the heat, cover and simmer for 30 minutes.

2. Add the garlic and bring to a boil again and then remove from the heat.

3. Transfer to a blender in batches and blend until smooth.

4. Serve with as much sauerkraut juice as tolerated. Some people start with a drop while others do ok with a teaspoon.

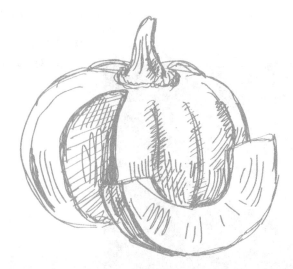

DINNER

GINGER LAMB SOUP

Serves: 4

Prep time: 15 minutes

Cook time: 25-30 minutes

Tip:

- Only lamb cooked in meat stock is ok at this stage.

Ingredients:

- 4 cups homemade stock
- 1 cup organic grass-fed lamb, cooked in meat stock
- 1 cup carrots, chopped
- ½ yellow onion, chopped
- 1 clove garlic, chopped
- Sauerkraut juice as tolerated

Directions:

1. Start by adding the lamb, carrots, and onion to a large stock pot with the meat stock and bring to a boil.

2. Reduce to a simmer and cook for 20-25 minutes or until the carrots and the chopped onion are tender.

3. Add the chopped garlic, bring to a boil again and then turn off the heat.

4. Serve with as much sauerkraut juice as tolerated. Some people start with a drop while others do ok with a teaspoon.

CHICKEN SQUASH SOUP

Serves: 4

Prep time: 15 minutes

Cook time: 25-30 minutes

Tip:

- Only chicken cooked as part of the meat stock making process is allowed at this stage.

Ingredients:

- 4 cups homemade stock
- 1 cup organic pasture-raised chicken, cooked in meat stock and shredded (You will want to use the meat that was cooked in the process of making homemade stock)
- 1 cup carrots, chopped
- ½ yellow onion, chopped
- ½ cup zucchini, peeled deseeded and grated
- 1 clove garlic, chopped
- Sauerkraut juice as tolerated

Directions:

1. Start by adding the chicken, carrots, zucchini and onion to a large stock pot with the meat stock and bring to a boil.

2. Reduce to a simmer and cook for 20-25 minutes or until the carrots, zucchini and the chopped onion is tender.

3. Add the chopped garlic, bring to a boil again and then turn off the heat.

4. Serve with as much sauerkraut juice as tolerated. Some people start with a drop while others do ok with a teaspoon.

BEEF SOUP

Serves: 4

Prep time: 15 minutes

Cook time: 30 minutes

Ingredients:

- 4 cups homemade stock
- 1 cup organic cooked grass-fed beef, cubed (you can use the beef cooked while making your homemade meat stock)
- 1 cup carrots, chopped
- ½ yellow onion, chopped
- 1 clove garlic, chopped
- Sauerkraut juice as tolerated

Directions:

1. Start by adding the carrots and onion to a large stock pot with meat stock and bring to a boil.

2. Reduce to a simmer and cook for 20-25 minutes or until the carrots and the chopped onion are tender.

3. Add the cooked cubed beef and onion, cook for an additional 5 minutes.

4. Serve with as much sauerkraut juice as tolerated. Some people start with a drop while others do ok with a teaspoon.

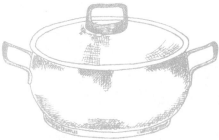

CHICKEN "NOODLE" SOUP

Serves: 4

Prep time: 15 minutes

Cook time: 30-35 minutes

Tip:

- Only chicken cooked while making meat stock is approved in this stage.

Ingredients:

- 4 cups homemade stock
- 1 cup organic pasture-raised chicken, cooked while making meat stock and shredded
- 1 cup carrots, chopped
- ½ yellow onion, chopped
- 1 zucchini, peeled and spiralized
- 1 clove garlic, chopped
- Sauerkraut juice as tolerated

Directions:

1. Start by adding the chicken, carrots, garlic, and onion to a large stock pot with the meat stock and bring to a boil.

2. Reduce to a simmer and cook for 20-25 minutes or until the carrots and the chopped onion is tender.

3. Add the zucchini and cook for another 5 minutes or until tender.

4. Serve with as much sauerkraut juice as tolerated. Some people start with a drop while others do ok with a teaspoon.

CARROT AND SQUASH BEEF SOUP

Serves: 4

Prep time: 15 minutes

Cook time: 25-30 minutes

Ingredients:

- 4 cups homemade stock
- 1 cup organic grass-fed beef, cubed
- 1 cup carrots, peeled and chopped
- ½ yellow onion, chopped
- 1 cup summer yellow squash, cubed
- 1 clove garlic, chopped
- Sauerkraut juice as tolerated

Directions:

1. Start by adding the beef, carrots, butternut squash and onion to a large stock pot with meat stock and bring to a boil.

2. Reduce to a simmer and cook for 20-25 minutes or until the carrots, butternut squash and the chopped onion are all tender and the beef is cooked through.

3. Add the chopped garlic, bring to a boil again and then turn off the heat.

4. Serve with as much sauerkraut juice as tolerated. Some people start with a drop while others do ok with a teaspoon.

SNACKS

MUG OF GINGER STOCK

Serves: 1

Prep time: 5 minutes

Cook time: 5 minutes

Ingredients:

- 1 cup homemade stock
- ½ tsp. fresh ginger, grated
- Pinch of mineral salt

Directions:

1. Simply add the homemade stock and ginger to a stockpot over medium heat and steep for at least three minutes.

2. Strain the ginger, and season with a pinch of mineral salt and enjoy right away.

HOMEMADE SOUR CREAM (AS TOLERATED)

Serves: 1

Prep time: 20 minutes

Cook time: 3-5 minutes + fermentation time (24 hours +)

Tip:
- If raw organic cream is used, skip the first two steps.

Ingredients:

- 1-quart organic grass-fed heavy cream
- ½ cup homemade yogurt or kefir

Directions:

1. Pour the cream into a pot and bring it to a boil, stirring constantly.

2. Take the pot off the heat, put a lid on top and place it in cold water to allow it to cool down more quickly.

3. Once the temperature of the cream has fallen to 105-113°F, pour the cream into mason jars and add the yogurt or kefir.

4. Place the jars into the oven with the oven lights on but do not turn the oven on.

5. Allow the jars to sit in the oven for at least 24 hours and then place in the refrigerator to set.

6. Enjoy as a dip with vegetables cooked in stock.

GINGER & RAW HONEY TEA

Serves: 1

Prep time: 5 minutes

Cook time: 7 minutes

Ingredients:

- 1 cup of filtered water
- 1 tsp. raw honey
- 1 tsp. fresh ginger, grated

Directions:

1. Start by bringing the filtered water to a boil.

2. Add the freshly grated ginger and simmer for 7 minutes.

3. Strain and then sweeten with raw honey.

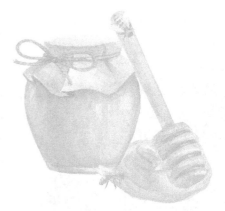

MINT TEA

Ingredients:

- 1 Tbsp. fresh mint leaves
- 8 ounces filtered water, hot
- ½ tsp. raw honey

Directions:

1. Place the mint leaves in a tea pot with the hot water.

2. Steep for 5 minutes before straining.

3. Sweeten with raw honey and enjoy right away.

Serves: 1

Prep time: 5 minutes

Cook time: 5 minutes

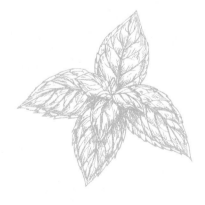

Stage 2

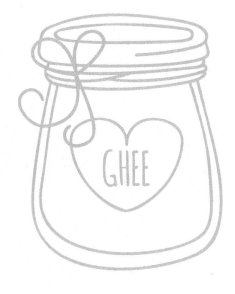

BREAKFAST

PORK BREAKFAST STEW

Serves: 4

Prep time: 15 minutes

Cook time: 30-35 minutes

Tip:

- Make a pork casserole for dinner the night before and use the leftover pork and stock for this recipe for breakfast!

Ingredients:

- 3 cups organic pasture-raised pork, cooked in meat stock and shredded (You will want to use the meat that was cooked in the process of making homemade stock)
- 2 cups homemade pork or chicken stock
- 2 zucchinis, peeled and chopped
- 1 tsp. fresh thyme, chopped
- 1 tsp. fresh rosemary, chopped
- Mineral salt to taste
- 1-2 Tbsp. duck or goose fat

Directions:

1. Melt the duck or goose fat in a large stock pot over medium heat.

2. Add the rest of the ingredients to the pot and cover with the stock.

3. Bring to a boil and then reduce the heat to low. Cook for about 25-30 minutes, until the vegetables are tender.

4. Serve hot and enjoy!

TURKEY BREAKFAST STEW

Serves: 4

Prep time: 15 minutes

Cook time: 30-35 minutes

Tip:

- Make a turkey casserole for dinner the night before and use the leftover turkey and stock for this recipe for breakfast!

Ingredients:

- 3 cups organic grass-fed ground turkey
- 1 leek, chopped
- 2 Tbsp. onion, chopped
- 2 cups homemade turkey or chicken stock
- 1 tsp. fresh thyme, chopped
- 1 tsp. fresh rosemary, chopped
- 1-2 Tbsp. duck or goose fat

Directions:

1. Melt the duck or goose fat in a large stock pot over medium heat.

2. Add the rest of the ingredients to the pot and cover with the stock.

3. Bring to a boil and then reduce the heat to low. Cook for about 30 minutes, until the vegetables are tender.

4. Serve hot and enjoy!

BREAKFAST SOUP

Serves: 1

Prep time: 5 minutes

Cook time: 5 minutes

Ingredients:

- 1 cup homemade stock
- 1 organic pasture-raised egg yolk
- 1 sprig fresh rosemary
- 2 Tbsp. onion, chopped
- 1 tsp. grass-fed ghee
- Mineral salt to taste

Directions:

1. Simply add all ingredients to a stock pot and whisk. Heat until warm and the egg yolk is cooked.

2. Remove the rosemary sprig before serving and enjoy.

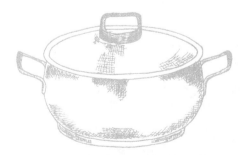

LUNCH

VEGETABLE CHICKEN STEW

Serves: 6

Prep time: 10 minutes

Cook time: 30 minutes

Ingredients:

- 2 lb. organic cooked pasture-raised chicken thighs (Use the meat that was previously cooked in the making of homemade stock)
- 2 cups homemade chicken stock
- 1 zucchini, peeled and chopped
- 1 small onion, chopped
- 1 clove garlic, chopped
- 4 carrots, peeled and chopped
- 1 tsp. mineral salt

Directions:

1. Add all of the ingredients to a large stock pot and cover with chicken stock.

2. Bring to a boil and then reduce the heat to low. Simmer for 30 minutes.

3. Stir and enjoy.

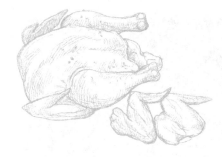

CARROT AND BEEF STEW

Serves: 6

Prep time: 10 minutes

Cook time: 50 minutes

Ingredients:

- 2 lb. organic grass-fed beef stew meat
- 2 cups filtered water
- 4 carrots, chopped
- 1 small onion, chopped
- 1 clove garlic, chopped
- 1 tsp. mineral salt

Directions:

1. Add all of the ingredients to a large stock pot and cover with the filtered water.

2. Bring to a boil and then reduce the heat to low. Simmer for 50 minutes or until the beef is cooked.

3. Serve hot.

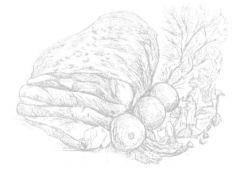

CROCKPOT CHICKEN AND PUMPKIN SOUP

Serves: 6

Prep time: 10 minutes

Cook time: 30 minutes

Ingredients:

- 2 lb. organic pasture-raised cooked chicken thighs (Use the meat that was cooked during the process of making homemade meatstock)
- 6 cups homemade chicken stock
- 1 cup pumpkin, peeled, seeded, and cubed
- 2 carrots, peeled and chopped
- 1 small onion, chopped
- 1 clove garlic, chopped
- 1 tsp. mineral salt

Directions:

1. Add all of the ingredients to a crockpot or slow cooker and cover with the chicken stock.

2. Simmer for 30 minutes.

3. Stir well and enjoy.

DINNER

CHICKEN PHO

Serves: 6

Prep time: 10 minutes

Cook time: 30 minutes

Ingredients:

- 4 cups homemade chicken stock
- 3 cups filtered water
- 2-inch piece of fresh ginger, sliced
- ½ tsp. mineral salt
- 2 cups organic pasture-raised chicken, cooked and shredded
- 1 large zucchini, peeled and spiralized
- 2 cloves garlic, chopped
- 1 cup fresh mixed herbs (basil, cilantro, parsley), chopped
- 1 organic pasture-raised egg yolk
- Sauerkraut juice as tolerated

Directions:

1. In a large pot, add the stock, water, ginger and salt. Bring to a boil, then reduce the heat to low and simmer for 15 minutes.

2. Add the chicken, zucchini, garlic and mixed herbs and simmer for 5-10 more minutes, or until zucchini is softened. Remove the fresh herbs and ginger.

3. Top with an egg yolk. Add a very small amount of sauerkraut juice to each serving once it has cooled enough to eat.

LAMB CASSEROLE WITH ROSEMARY

Serves: 10

Prep time: 10 minutes

Cook time: 5-6 hours

Ingredients:

- 5 lb. organic grass-fed leg of lamb
- Filtered water
- 1 tsp. mineral salt
- 1 Tbsp. peppercorns, crushed (in a cache to easily remove)
- 2 bay leaves
- 1 sprig of fresh rosemary
- 3 or 4 small red onions, peeled
- 2 cups broccoli florets
- 2 cups cauliflower florets
- 3 or 4 carrots, chopped into large pieces

Directions:

1. Preheat the oven to 300F.

2. Add the leg of lamb to a large casserole dish with a lid and pour the filtered water into the dish until it is about two thirds full. Add the salt, peppercorns, bay leaves and rosemary. Cover with the lid and put it in the oven for 5-6 hours.

3. After 4-5 hours of cooking, add the red onions, broccoli, cauliflower and carrots.

4. Once cooked, remove the herbs and peppercorn.

5. Place the leg of lamb and vegetables on a serving dish ready to be served up.

6. Sieve the meat stock left in the casserole dish and serve with dinner in bouillon cups or small bowls.

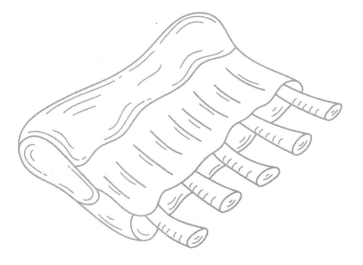

SQUASH AND GROUND BEEF MASH

Serves: 4

Prep time: 10 minutes

Cook time: 30 minutes

Tip:

- The drained stock can be enjoyed as a hot drink alongside the mash.

Ingredients:

- 1 lb. organic grass-fed ground beef
- 1 onion, chopped
- 2 cloves garlic, chopped
- 1 tsp. mineral salt
- 1 lb. yellow summer squash, peeled and chopped into small pieces
- 2 Tbsp. grass-fed ghee, melted
- 4 cups homemade stock

Directions:

1. In a bowl, mix together the beef, onion, garlic and half a teaspoon of salt.

2. Add the squash to the melted ghee and the remaining half teaspoon of salt in a large stock pot and toss to combine.

3. Scoop the ground beef on top of the squash and pour the stock over top. Bring to a boil over high heat, then reduce the heat to low, cover and simmer for 25 minutes, or until the squash and beef are cooked through.

4. Drain any stock remaining after cooking and use a potato masher to mash everything up.

SNACKS

SOFT-BOILED EGG YOLKS

Serves: 3

Prep time: 5 minutes

Cook time: 10 minutes

Ingredients:

- 3 organic pasture-raised eggs
- 1 pinch of mineral salt

Directions:

1. Bring a large pot of water to a boil and boil the eggs for about 10 minutes.

2. Allow the eggs to cool and then remove the egg whites.

3. Season the soft-boiled egg yolk with mineral salt and enjoy as a quick snack.

4. Make a few ahead of time to always have on hand when you get hungry and need a quick and easy snack.

CUBED PUMPKIN WITH SEA SALT

Serves: 4

Prep Time: 10 minutes

Cook Time: 30 minutes

Ingredients:

- 1 pumpkin, skin removed and cubed
- 1 pinch of mineral salt
- Meat stock for cooking

Directions:

1. Start by cooking the cubed pumpkin in meat stock until tender, this should take about 30 minutes.

2. Once cooked, serve the cubed pumpkin with a pinch of mineral salt.

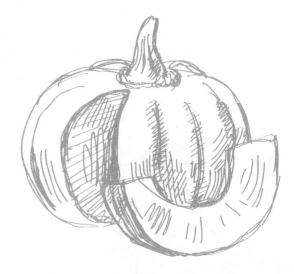

KEFIR (AS TOLERATED)

Serves: 4

Prep time: 24-27 hours

Cook time: 0 minutes

Tip:

- Where possible, use raw organic milk as this is much richer in nutrients since it has not been pasteurized or processed.

Ingredients:

- 2 Tbsp. kefir grains
- 2 cups raw organic milk

Directions:

1. Start by adding the kefir grains to the base of a large glass jar and cover with milk.

2. Swirl to mix and then cover the jar and allow it to sit at room temperature for 24-27 hours.

3. Strain the kefir to remove the grains, using a fine mesh strainer or colander placed over a large bowl. The mixture should be thick so you will likely need to use a spoon to press down on the strainer or colander to separate more kefir from the grains.

4. Once you are just left with the liquid, transfer it to a large glass jar.

5. Enjoy! Store leftovers in the refrigerator.

Stage 3

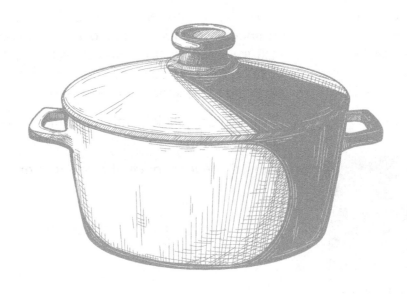

BREAKFAST

HERBY SCRAMBLED EGGS WITH SAUERKRAUT

Serves: 2

Prep time: 10 minutes

Cook time: 15-20 minutes

Ingredients:

- 4 organic pasture-raised eggs
- ½ cup fresh parsley, chopped
- ¼ tsp. mineral salt
- 3 Tbsp. grass-fed ghee
- 1 small onion, chopped
- Sauerkraut juice as tolerated

Directions:

1. In a small bowl, whisk together the eggs, parsley and salt

2. In a large skillet, melt the ghee over medium heat. Add the onion, cover and cook on low for 10 minutes, or until the onions are soft.

3. Add the egg mixture to the skillet and cook on low, stirring occasionally, until the eggs are cooked.

4. Serve with as much sauerkraut juice as tolerated. Some people start with a drop while others do ok with a teaspoon.

61

BREAKFAST MASH BOWL

Serves: 2

Prep time: 10 minutes

Cook time: 40 minutes

Tip:

- Be careful that the mash does not burn on the bottom while the eggs are cooking.

Ingredients:

- 1 cup homemade stock
- 1 lb. pumpkin, peeled, seeded, and cut into cubes
- 1 onion, chopped
- 4 cloves garlic, chopped
- ½ tsp. mineral salt
- 4 organic pasture-raised eggs
- ¼ avocado

Directions:

1. In a large pot, add the stock, pumpkin, onion and garlic. Cover and simmer for 30 minutes or until the squash is completely cooked through.

2. Once cooked, add the salt and use a potato masher or fork to mash everything together.

3. Crack the eggs on top of the mash, cover and cook over low heat for 10 more minutes, or until the eggs are cooked through.

4. Serve warm topped with avocado.

THAI PEANUT BUTTER PANCAKES

Serves: 1-2

Prep time: 10 minutes

Cook time: 10-15 minutes

Ingredients:

- ½ cup pumpkin, steamed and mashed
- ¼ cup fresh basil, chopped
- 3 Tbsp. organic peanut butter
- 2 organic pasture-raised eggs
- ¼ tsp. mineral salt
- 3 Tbsp. grass-fed ghee

Directions:

1. In a bowl, mix together the pumpkin, basil, peanut butter, eggs and salt.

2. In a large skillet, melt the ghee over medium-low heat. Scoop the batter into the pan to form small pancakes.

3. Cook for about 2-3 minutes per side, being careful not to let it burn.

4. Enjoy warm, topped with more ghee if desired.

LUNCH

CREAMY CAULIFLOWER SOUP

Serves: 2

Prep time: 10 minutes

Cook time: 30 minutes + thickening time (20 minutes +)

Tip:
- Add some mashed avocado to the soup for added flavor and texture.

Ingredients:

- ¼ cup grass-fed ghee
- 1 head cauliflower, cut into florets
- 1 onion, chopped
- 5 cups homemade stock
- ¼ tsp. mineral salt
- ¼ tsp. black pepper, freshly ground
- Sauerkraut juice as tolerated

Directions:

1. In a large pot, melt the ghee over medium heat.

2. Add the onions, cauliflower, stock, salt and pepper. Cover and simmer for 30 minutes or until the cauliflower is cooked through.

3. Purée in a blender or with an immersion stick until smooth. Allow to sit for at least 20 minutes to let the soup thicken up and become creamy.

4. Serve with as much sauerkraut juice as tolerated. Some people start with a drop while others do ok with a teaspoon.

MEATBALL MINESTRONE

Serves: 2-3

Prep time: 10 minutes

Cook time: 30 minutes

Ingredients:

- 1 lb. organic grass-fed ground beef
- ½ cup fresh parsley, chopped
- 1 egg
- ½ tsp. mineral salt
- ¼ cup grass-fed ghee
- 1 onion
- 2 cups cauliflower florets
- 4 cups homemade stock
- Sauerkraut juice as tolerated

Directions:

1. To make the meatballs, mix the beef, parsley, egg and salt together in a medium bowl. Form into small meatballs and set aside.

2. In a large pot, melt the ghee over medium heat.

3. Add the onions, cauliflower, meatballs and stock. Bring to a boil, then reduce the heat to low and simmer for 30 minutes or until the meatballs are cooked through and the cauliflower is soft.

4. Enjoy warm, topped with as much sauerkraut juice as tolerated. Some people start with a drop while others do ok with a teaspoon.

CREAMY SALMON DILL SALAD

Serves: 4

Prep time: 10 minutes

Cook time: 10-15 minutes

Ingredients:

- 4 cups filtered water
- 1 lb. wild salmon
- ½ avocado, mashed
- ½ cup fresh dill
- 2 Tbsp. homemade yogurt (if tolerated)
- 2 Tbsp. lemon juice
- 2 Tbsp. fish stock
- ½ tsp. mineral salt

Directions:

1. In a large pot, bring 4 cups of water to a boil. Add the salmon to the pot and boil for about 10-12 minutes, or until the salmon is cooked through.

2. Remove the salmon from the pot and place in a large bowl. Add the avocado, dill, yogurt (if using), lemon juice, fish stock, and mineral salt.

3. Mash and mix the ingredients together until everything is combined. Enjoy with a warm mug of homemade stock.

ASIAN BOK CHOY AND CAULI-RICE

Serves: 4

Prep time: 10 minutes

Cook time: 10 minutes

Ingredients:

- ½ cup homemade fish stock
- 1 head cauliflower, cut into florets
- 1 Tbsp. fresh ginger, grated
- 2 Tbsp. lime juice
- 2 Tbsp. grass-fed ghee
- ¼ tsp. mineral salt
- 2 heads bok choy, sliced into quarters lengthwise
- 2 cups organic pasture-raised chicken, cooked and shredded (cooked in meat stock)

Directions:

1. Add the cauliflower to a food processor and pulse until it starts to resemble rice.

2. In a large skillet, heat the stock over medium heat. Once it starts to simmer, add the cauliflower and the shredded chicken. Cover and let it cook for 5 minutes, or until the cauliflower is cooked.

3. Remove from the heat and mix in the ginger, lime juice, ghee and salt. Transfer to a bowl.

4. In the same skillet, add the bok choy and a bit of water to steam the bok choy for 3-5 minutes.

5. Serve the bok choy with the shredded chicken and cauli-rice.

67

DINNER

SPRING ASPARAGUS AND ZUCCHINI SOUP

Serves: 4

Prep time: 10 minutes

Cook time: 20 minutes + cooling time (1 hour)

Ingredients:

- 4 cups homemade stock
- 1 bunch asparagus, ends removed
- 1 large zucchini, sliced
- 2 cloves garlic, chopped
- ½ tsp. mineral salt
- 1 Tbsp. lemon juice
- 2 raw egg yolks

Directions:

1. In a large pot, bring the stock to a boil. Add the asparagus, zucchini, garlic and salt. Cover and then simmer for 20 minutes or until the vegetables are cooked through.

2. Allow the soup to cool for an hour, then pour into a blender (or use an immersion stick) with the lemon juice and egg yolks and blend until smooth.

3. Serve cold or heat the soup up over a low heat before serving.

GINGER BEEF AND BROCCOLI

Serves: 4

Prep time: 10 minutes

Cook time: 20-25 minutes

Ingredients:

- 2 Tbsp. grass-fed ghee
- 1 onion, chopped
- 2 cups homemade beef stock
- 2-inch piece fresh ginger, chopped
- 2 cloves garlic, chopped
- 1 lb. organic grass-fed ground beef
- 1 head broccoli, cut into florets
- ½ tsp. mineral salt
- ¼ cup fresh cilantro, chopped
- ½ avocado, sliced
- Sauerkraut juice as tolerated

Directions:

1. In a large skillet, melt the ghee over medium heat. Add the onion and cook until softened, for about 10 minutes.

2. Add the stock, ginger, garlic, ground beef, broccoli and salt.

3. Use a spoon to break up the ground beef. Cover and bring to a simmer. Let everything cook for 10-15 minutes, or until the beef is cooked through and broccoli is soft.

4. Top with cilantro, and avocado.

5. Serve with as much sauerkraut juice as tolerated. Some people start with a drop while others do ok with a teaspoon.

CHICKEN AND CAULI-TABBOULEH

Serves: 4

Prep time: 10 minutes

Cook time: 5 minutes

Ingredients:

- 1 head cauliflower, cut into florets
- ¼ cup + 2 Tbsp. homemade chicken stock
- ½ cup fresh mint, chopped
- ½ cup fresh parsley, chopped
- ½ cup fresh basil, chopped
- 2 tsp. lemon juice
- ½ tsp. mineral salt
- 2 cups chicken, cooked and shredded (cooked in meatstock)
- ¼ avocado, sliced

Directions:

1. In a food processor, pulse the cauliflower until it resembles rice.

2. In a large skillet, heat a quarter cup of stock. Add the cauliflower rice and cook, covered, for 5 minutes or until softened and liquid has evaporated.

3. Pour the cauliflower rice into a bowl and mix in the remaining 2 tablespoons of stock, mint, parsley, basil, lemon juice and salt.

4. Serve the cauli-tabbouleh topped with the shredded chicken and avocado.

ROASTED CHICKEN WITH CILANTRO LIME CAULI-RICE

Serves: 4

Prep time: 15 minutes

Cook time: 5-10 minutes

Ingredients:

- ½ cup homemade chicken stock
- 1 head cauliflower, cut into florets
- ½ cup fresh cilantro, chopped
- 2 Tbsp. lime juice
- Sauerkraut juice as tolerated
- 2 Tbsp. grass-fed ghee
- ¼ tsp. mineral salt
- 2 cups organic pasture-raised chicken, cooked and shredded (cooked in meat stock)
- 1 organic and pasture-raised egg yolk

Directions:

1. Add the cauliflower to a food processor and pulse until it starts to resemble rice.

2. In a large skillet, heat the stock over medium heat. Once it starts to simmer, add the cauliflower. Cover and let cook for 5 minutes or until the cauliflower is cooked.

71

3. Remove from the heat and mix in the cilantro, lime juice, ghee and salt.

4. Add as much sauerkraut juice as tolerated. Some people start with a drop while others do ok with a teaspoon.

5. Top with the shredded chicken and an egg yolk.

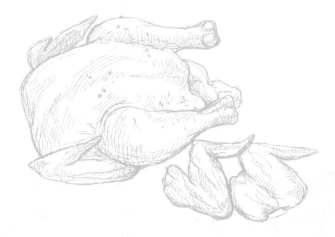

SNACKS

MINI PUMPKIN PANCAKES

Serves: 1

Prep time: 5 minutes

Cook time: 12-15 minutes

Ingredients:

- 3 Tbsp. grass-fed ghee
- ½ cup pumpkin, steamed and mashed
- 2 Tbsp. organic almond butter
- 2 organic pasture-raised egg yolks

Directions:

1. In a small bowl, whisk together the pumpkin, almond butter and egg yolks.

2. In a large skillet, heat the ghee over medium heat. Spoon a small amount of the batter into the hot pan to make a mini pancake. Cook until golden brown, for about 3 minutes, being careful not to let it burn.

3. Flip and cook for an additional 3 minutes.

4. Make a further 2-3 mini pancakes until the mixture is all used up.

5. Enjoy hot or store in the refrigerator or freezer and pop in the toaster for an on-the-go snack.

AVOCADO AND SAUERKRAUT

Serves: 1

Prep time: 5 minutes

Cook time: 0 minutes

Tip:

- The recipe for homemade sauerkraut can be found in the base recipes section.

Ingredients:

- ¼ avocado, pitted and mashed
- Sauerkraut as tolerated
- 1 pinch of Celtic sea salt

Directions:

1. Slice the avocado and mash with the sauerkraut. Some people start with a drop while others do ok with a teaspoon.

2. Season with salt and enjoy right away.

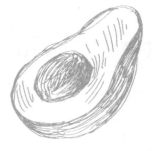

ONION EGG SCRAMBLE

Serves: 2

Prep time: 5 minutes

Cook time: 25 minutes

Ingredients:

- 4 organic pasture-raised eggs, whisked
- ¼ cup white onion, chopped
- 4 Tbsp. grass-fed ghee
- Pinch of mineral salt

Directions:

1. Start by heating the ghee in a pan over low heat and add the onion. Cover the pan and cook for about 20 minutes.

2. Add the eggs and scramble until cooked. Mix the onions in well whilst stirring.

3. Serve with a pinch of salt and enjoy.

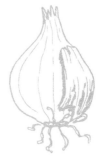

LACTO-FERMENTED CARROTS

Serves: 12

Prep time: 10 minutes + fermentation time (7 days)

Cook time: 0 minutes

Ingredients:

- 2 cups filtered water
- 2 lb. carrots, sliced
- 1½ Tbsp. mineral salt
- 2 Tbsp. fresh dill, chopped

Directions:

1. Start by dissolving the salt in the 2 cups of water in a large mixing bowl.

2. Add the carrots to a mason style glass jar and fill with the water.

3. Add the fresh dill to the jar.

4. Cover the jar and allow it to sit for 2 days. After two days, carefully release some of the air from the jar by unscrewing the cap and letting just a small amount of air out. This is called "burping"

5. Allow the carrots to ferment for about 7 days, "burping" the jars every couple of days.

6. Store the carrots in the refrigerator and enjoy as an easy on-the-go snack.

FAT BOMBS

Serves: 3

Prep time: 5 minutes + chilling time (1 hour)

Cook time: 5 minutes

Ingredients:

- 1 Tbsp. grass-fed ghee
- 1 Tbsp. raw honey
- 1/8 tsp. fresh ginger, grated

Directions:

1. Start by adding the ghee to a stockpot over low heat and stir to combine. Remove from heat.

2. Add in the ginger, and honey and stir.

3. Pour the mixture into molds, adding 1 teaspoon of the mixture to each mold and refrigerate for 1 hour before enjoying.

4. Store any leftovers in the refrigerator.

Stage 4

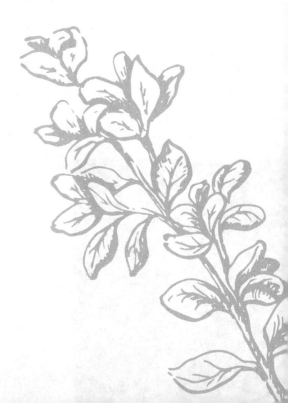

BREAKFAST

GREEN FRITTATA

Serves: 4

Prep time: 10 minutes

Cook time: 30 minutes

Ingredients:

- 8 organic pasture-raised eggs
- ¼ cup homemade yogurt
- 1 tsp. dried oregano
- ½ cup fresh parsley, chopped
- 2 Tbsp. grass-fed ghee
- ½ small onion, sliced
- ½ tsp. mineral salt
- 1 bunch asparagus
- 2 cloves garlic, minced

Directions:

1. Preheat the oven to 325°F.

2. In a large bowl, whisk together the eggs, yogurt, oregano and parsley. Set aside.

3. In a large ovenproof skillet (cast-iron is best), heat the ghee over medium heat. Add the onion and sauté until it begins to brown, for about 10 minutes.

4. Add the asparagus and garlic and cook, stirring frequently, for about 1 minute.

5. Pour the egg mixture into the pan and cook over medium heat for 5 minutes, or until the edges begin to set.

6. Transfer to the oven and bake for about 15 minutes, or until the eggs have set in the center. Cut into 8 slices and eat right away or let them cool completely and store them in the refrigerator.

CAULI 'OATMEAL'

Serves: 4

Prep time: 15 minutes

Cook time: 5 minutes

Ingredients:

- 2 Tbsp. grass-fed ghee
- 1 head cauliflower, cut into florets
- 2 Tbsp. fresh ginger, grated
- 1 Tbsp. raw honey
- 1 Tbsp. almond butter
- ¼ tsp. mineral salt

Directions:

1. Add the cauliflower to a food processor and pulse until it starts to resemble rice.

2. In a large skillet, melt the ghee over medium heat. Add the cauliflower, cover and let it cook for 5 minutes.

3. Stir in the ginger, honey, almond butter and salt.

AVOCADO LIME SMOOTHIE

Serves: 1

Prep time: 10 minutes

Cook time: 0 minutes

Ingredients:

- 1 cup homemade stock
- 1 cup filtered water
- ¼ avocado
- 1 Tbsp. almond butter
- 1 Tbsp. lime juice
- 2 tsp. raw honey

Directions:

1. Add all of the ingredients to a high-speed blender and blend until smooth. If the smoothie is too thick, add more water.

2. Pour into a glass and enjoy!

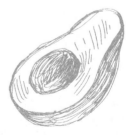

LUNCH

AVOCADO EGG SALAD

Serves: 2

Prep time: 10 minutes

Cook time: 0 minutes

Tip:
- Leave the yogurt out if dairy is not tolerated.

Ingredients:

- 4 organic pasture-raised eggs, hard-boiled
- ½ avocado
- ¼ cup fresh herbs, chopped
- 2 Tbsp. homemade yogurt
- 1 Tbsp. lemon or lime juice
- ¼ tsp. mineral salt
- ¼ tsp. black pepper, freshly ground

Directions:

1. In a small bowl, add the eggs and avocado. Using a fork, mash the eggs and avocado until they are all broken up.

2. Add the herbs, yogurt (if using), lemon or lime juice, salt and pepper.

3. Enjoy on top of a slice of almond flour bread.

ROASTED CHICKEN WITH SQUASH FRIES

Serves: 4

Prep time: 10 minutes

Cook time: 20 minutes

Ingredients:

- 1 lb. organic pasture-raised chicken thighs
- Salt and pepper to taste
- 1 medium yellow summer squash, peeled and cut into fries
- 2 Tbsp. grass-fed ghee, melted
- 1 tsp. garlic powder
- ½ tsp. mineral salt

Directions:

1. Preheat the oven to 350°F. Line a standard baking sheet with parchment paper.

2. Place the chicken thighs on half of the baking sheet and sprinkle generously with salt and pepper.

3. In a large bowl, mix together the squash, ghee, garlic powder and half teaspoon of salt. Pour the fries onto the other half of the baking sheet

4. Bake for 10 minutes, flip the fries and bake for another 10 minutes or until the chicken and squash are both cooked through.

ASPARAGUS AND MINT SOUP

Serves: 4

Prep time: 10 minutes

Cook time: 20 minutes

Ingredients:

- 2 Tbsp. grass-fed ghee
- 1 onion, chopped
- 1 bunch asparagus
- ½ tsp. mineral salt
- 2 cloves garlic, chopped
- 4 cups homemade stock
- ½ cup fresh parsley, chopped
- ½ cup fresh basil, chopped
- 1 Tbsp. cold-pressed olive oil

Directions:

1. In a large pot, melt the ghee over medium heat. Add the onions, asparagus and salt. Cook for 5 minutes, stirring occasionally, until the onions soften.

2. Add the garlic and stock, cover and simmer for 15 minutes.

3. Pour the soup into a blender with the parsley and basil. Blend until smooth.

4. Serve warm with the olive oil drizzled on top.

LEMON AND HERB ROASTED SALMON AND CARROTS

Serves: 4

Prep time: 10 minutes

Cook time: 12 minutes

Ingredients:

- 1 lb. wild salmon
- ¼ cup fresh parsley, chopped
- 1 lemon, sliced
- 3 Tbsp. grass-fed ghee
- 4 large carrots, sliced
- 1 Tbsp. grass-fed ghee, melted
- ¼ tsp. mineral salt

Directions:

1. Preheat the oven to 350°F. Line a baking sheet with parchment paper.

2. Place the salmon fillets on the baking sheet. Season with salt and pepper. Top with the parsley, lemon slices and 3 tablespoons of ghee.

3. Add the carrots to the baking sheet and toss with the melted ghee and salt.

4. Bake for 12 minutes, or until the salmon is cooked through.

85

GREEN EGGS ON TOAST

Serves: 1

Prep time: 5 minutes

Cook time: 15 minutes

Tip:

- The recipe for homemade almond bread can be found below under 'SNACKS' for this stage.

Ingredients:

- 1 slice homemade almond bread
- 2 Tbsp. grass-fed ghee
- ½ onion
- ¼ tsp. mineral salt
- 1 cup fresh spinach
- 2 organic pasture-raised eggs

Directions:

1. In a skillet, warm the ghee over medium heat. Add the onions and salt and cook on low until softened, about 10 minutes. Add the spinach and eggs and cook, stirring to scramble the eggs, until the eggs are cooked through.

2. Toast the almond bread in a toaster or under the grill.

3. Serve the eggs on top of the toasted bread.

DINNER

MEXICAN BEEF PATTIES WITH AVOCADO MASH

Serves: 4

Prep time: 10 minutes

Cook time: 15-20 minutes

Ingredients:

- 1 lb. organic grass-fed ground beef
- ¼ cup homemade almond flour
- 1 cup fresh parsley, chopped
- 1 organic pasture-raised egg
- 1 tsp. mineral salt
- 2 Tbsp. grass-fed ghee

- Filtered water
- 3 cups broccoli florets
- 2 avocados, pitted and peeled
- 2 Tbsp. lime juice
- Homemade sauerkraut as tolerated

Directions:

1. In a large bowl, mix together the ground beef, almond flour, half a cup of parsley, egg and half a teaspoon of salt. Form into 4 large patties, putting a slight indentation in the center of each patty to keep it from swelling up during cooking.

2. Grill the patties under medium heat for 5 minutes on each side, or until well done and cooked through.

3. In a medium pot, bring 1-inch of water to a simmer over low heat. Add the broccoli, cover and steam for 5-7 minutes, or until very soft and easy to mash.

4. In a medium bowl, mash together the steamed broccoli, avocado, lime juice, remaining half cup of parsley and remaining half a teaspoon of salt.

5. Serve the burgers topped with the avocado mash and sauerkraut. Serve with as much sauerkraut as tolerated. Some people start with a drop while others do ok with a teaspoon.

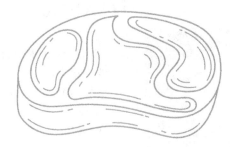

ROASTED CHICKEN WITH CILANTRO LIME SAUCE

Serves: 4

Prep time: 10 minutes

Cook time: 30 minutes

Ingredients:

- 1 lb. organic pasture-raised chicken thighs (skin left on, bone left in)
- 1 head cauliflower, cut into small florets
- 3 Tbsp. coconut oil, melted
- ¼ tsp. mineral salt
- ¼ tsp. black pepper, freshly ground

- Cilantro Lime Sauce:
- 2 cups fresh cilantro, finely chopped
- ½ cup cold-pressed olive oil
- 1 Tbsp. lime juice
- 1 tsp. garlic powder
- ½ tsp. Celtic sea salt
- ¼ tsp. black pepper, freshly ground

Directions:

1. Preheat the oven to 350°F. Line a standard baking sheet with parchment paper.

2. Place the chicken thighs on half of the baking sheet and the cauliflower on the other half. Drizzle the chicken and cauliflower with the coconut oil.

3. Bake for 30 minutes, or until the chicken and cauliflower are cooked through.

4. To make the sauce, add the cilantro, olive oil, lime juice, garlic powder, salt and pepper to a small bowl and whisk vigorously to combine.

5. Serve the chicken and cauliflower topped with the cilantro lime sauce.

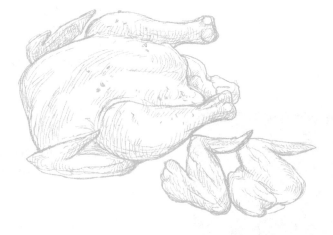

HERBED ROASTED SALMON AND ASPARAGUS

Serves: 4

Prep time: 10 minutes

Cook time: 12 minutes

Ingredients:

- 1 lb. wild salmon filets
- 1 bunch asparagus
- ½ cup grass-fed ghee
- 2 Tbsp. dried basil
- 1 Tbsp. dried oregano
- ½ tsp. mineral salt

Directions:

1. Preheat the oven to 350°F. Line a standard baking sheet with parchment paper.

2. Place the salmon on one half of the baking sheet and the asparagus on the other half.

3. To make the herbed ghee, add the ghee, basil, oregano and salt to a small bowl. Use a fork to mash everything together.

4. Divide the ghee evenly on top of the salmon and asparagus. Bake for 12 minutes, or until the salmon is cooked through.

SNACKS

GAPS GRANOLA

Serves: 6

Prep time: 5 minutes

Cook time: 10 minutes

Ingredients:

- 4 Tbsp. pecans
- 4 Tbsp. almonds
- 4 Tbsp. pumpkin seeds
- ¼ cup coconut oil, melted

Directions:

1. Start by preheating the oven to 300°F and line a baking sheet with parchment paper.

2. Add the nuts and coconut oil to a large bowl and toss to combine.

3. Transfer the nuts to the baking sheet and bake for 10 minutes or until lightly toasted.

4. Enjoy as an easy snack or serve with a cup of homemade yogurt.

CARROT JUICE

Serves: 4

Prep time: 10 minutes

Cook time: 0 minutes

Tip:

- If you do not have a juicer, you can make the juice in a high-speed blender and then strain the juice using a fine mesh strainer after blending.

Ingredients:

- 2 cups carrots

Directions:

1. Run the carrots through a juicer and then strain using a fine mesh strainer to make sure that the juice is clear and filtered.

2. Enjoy, starting with only a few spoonful's at a time.

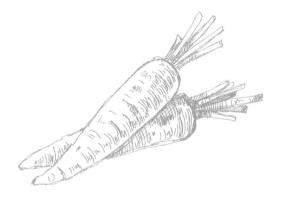

CELERY MINT JUICE

Serves: 4

Prep time: 10 minutes

Cook time: 0 minutes

Tip:

- If you do not have a juicer, you can make the juice in a high-speed blender and then strain the juice using a fine mesh strainer after blending.

- Only add this juice to your diet once you have introduced and tolerated carrot juice. This juice should be consumed on an empty stomach - for example, before breakfast.

Ingredients:

- 1 bunch celery stalks, washed
- 1 handful fresh mint leaves
- 1 cup filtered water

Directions:

1. Run the celery and mint leaves through a juicer and then strain using a fine mesh strainer to make sure that the juice is clear and filtered.

2. Dilute with water and enjoy!

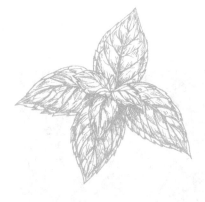

94

ALMOND FLOUR BREAD

Serves: 8

Prep time: 15 minutes

Cook time: 45-60 minutes

Tip:

- To make your own homemade almond flour, simply add almonds to a coffee grinder or food processor and blend until a flour-like consistency forms.

Ingredients:

- 2 cups homemade almond flour
- 2 organic pasture-raised eggs
- 1½ cups zucchini, grated
- 2 Tbsp. softened coconut oil + extra for greasing
- 1 Tbsp. grass-fed ghee

Directions:

1. Start by preheating the oven to 350°F and greasing a loaf pan with coconut oil.

2. Add all the ingredients to a bowl and stir to combine.

3. Pour the mixture into the loaf pan and press the mixture down into the pan.

4. Bake for 45-60 minutes or until a knife inserted into the center comes out clean.

5. Allow the bread to cool before slicing.

6. Enjoy with a teaspoon of ghee or coconut oil, if desired.

Stage 5

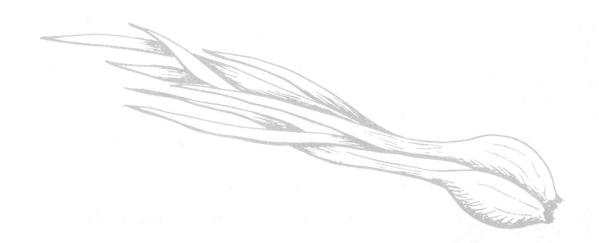

BREAKFAST

BREAKFAST APPLESAUCE

Serves: 2

Prep time: 10 minutes

Cook time: 15 minutes

Ingredients:

- 2 ripe apples peeled, cored and chopped
- ¼ cup homemade stock
- ¼ tsp. ground cinnamon
- ½ Tbsp. grass-fed ghee
- Drizzle of raw honey

Directions:

1. Start by coring, peeling and chopping the apples and adding them to a stockpot with the stock and cinnamon.

2. Bring to a simmer and cook for about 15 minutes or until the apples are tender.

3. Stir in the ghee and divide into 2 servings.

4. Drizzle with raw honey and enjoy right away.

EGG FRITTATA

Serves: 8

Prep time: 10 minutes

Cook time: 15-20 minutes

Tip:

- If you have any issues with nightshades, omit the tomatoes from the recipe and go back to previous stages.

Ingredients:

- 10 organic pasture-raised eggs
- 1 onion, chopped
- 2 tomatoes, chopped
- ¼ cup mushrooms, chopped
- 1 cup fresh spinach
- 4 Tbsp. grass-fed ghee
- Celtic sea salt and black pepper, freshly ground, to taste

Directions:

1. Start by adding the eggs, salt and pepper to a large mixing bowl and whisk well.

2. Heat a large skillet over medium heat with the ghee and pour in the egg mixture.

3. Add the rest of the ingredients to the skillet and cook until set.

4. Remove from the heat and cover and then let the eggs continue to set until completely set.

5. Serve hot or cold. Refrigerate any leftovers.

EGG MUFFINS

Serves: 12

Prep time: 10 minutes

Cook time: 12-15 minutes

Ingredients:

- 12 organic pasture-raised eggs
- 1 onion, chopped
- 1 clove garlic, chopped
- 1 cup broccoli, chopped
- 1 tomato, chopped
- 4 Tbsp. grass-fed ghee for greasing
- Green onion, chopped, for topping

Directions:

1. Start by preheating the oven to 400°F and greasing a muffin tin with ghee.

2. Add the eggs and all of the other ingredients, minus the ghee and green onion, to a large mixing bowl and whisk well.

3. Pour the egg mixture into the muffin tins and bake for about 12-15 minutes or until the muffins are completely cooked through.

4. Top with chopped green onion once cooked and store leftovers in the refrigerator for an easy grab-and-go breakfast.

LUNCH

MEAT ROLL UPS

Serves: 1

Prep time: 10 minutes

Cook time: 0 minutes

Tip:

- Pin each slice with a cocktail stick once filled if not enjoying straightaway. Refrigerate any leftovers.

- If you have any issues with nightshades, omit the tomatoes from the recipe. Cooked and peeled beetroot may be used instead of tomatoes.

Ingredients:

- 2 thick slices organic pasture-raised turkey breast, cooked
- 2 lettuce leaves
- 2 slices of tomato
- ¼ avocado, sliced
- Sauerkraut as tolerated

Directions:

1. Start by laying the turkey breast slices out onto a plate and evenly split the filling ingredients between the two slices.

2. Fill each piece of turkey breast with the lettuce leaf, tomato, avocado and sauerkraut. Serve with as much sauerkraut as tolerated. Some people start with a drop while others do ok with a teaspoon.

3. Roll up into a wrap and enjoy.

CAULIFLOWER RICE

Serves: 2

Prep time: 15 minutes

Cook time: 5-7 minutes

Ingredients:

- 1 head organic cauliflower, chopped
- ¼ cup homemade stock
- ¼ cup cabbage, chopped
- 1 carrot, chopped
- 1 small onion, chopped
- 1 clove garlic, chopped
- 1 Tbsp. fresh parsley, chopped
- Mineral salt and black pepper, freshly ground, to taste

Directions:

1. Start by adding the chopped cauliflower to a food processor and pulse until a rice-like consistency forms.

2. Add in the cabbage, carrots, onion, garlic and parsley and pulse for another 5-10 seconds or until combined.

3. Add the stock to a large skillet and add the cauliflower mixture. Sauté for about 5-7 minutes or until all the vegetables are tender and the stock has cooked down.

4. Season with salt and pepper and enjoy.

BEEF SALAD

Serves: 2

Prep time: 10 minutes

Cook time: 0 minutes

Ingredients:

- ½ lb. organic grass-fed beef, cooked and thinly sliced
- 2 cups lettuce, chopped or sliced
- 1 Tbsp. fresh rosemary, chopped
- 2 Tbsp. cold-pressed olive oil
- Mineral salt and black pepper, freshly ground, to taste
- Sauerkraut for serving

Directions:

1. Season the beef with 1 tablespoon of olive oil, rosemary, salt and pepper.

2. Serve the cooked beef on a bed of lettuce, with an extra drizzle of olive oil and some sauerkraut, if desired.

CUCUMBER AND AVOCADO SALAD

Serves: 2

Prep time: 10 minutes

Cook time: 0 minutes

Tip:

- Leave the yogurt out if dairy is not tolerated.

Ingredients:

- 2 Tbsp. cold-pressed olive oil
- 1 Tbsp. homemade yogurt
- 1 Tbsp. lemon juice
- ½ tsp. mineral salt
- 2 large cucumbers, peeled and sliced
- 1 avocado, chopped into bite-sized pieces
- 1 head butter lettuce, tough parts removed and chopped
- ¼ cup fresh dill, chopped

Directions:

1. In a large bowl, whisk together the olive oil, yogurt (if using), lemon juice and salt.

2. Add the cucumbers, avocado, lettuce and dill and toss to combine.

3. Enjoy straight away.

DINNER

ROASTED CHICKEN AND VEGGIES WITH CHIMICHURRI

Serves: 3

Prep time: 15 minutes

Cook time: 30-45 minutes

Ingredients:

- 1 lb. pumpkin, peeled and cut into cubes
- 1 head broccoli, cut into florets
- 2 Tbsp. coconut oil, melted
- ¼ tsp. mineral salt
- 6 organic pasture-fed chicken thighs
- For the chimichurri:

- 2 cups fresh parsley, chopped
- 2 cloves garlic, minced
- 2 Tbsp. lemon juice, freshly squeezed
- ¼ - ½ cup cold-pressed olive oil
- Celtic sea salt and black pepper, freshly ground, to taste

Directions:

1. Start by preheating the oven to 400°F and lining a baking sheet with parchment paper.

2. Add the pumpkin and broccoli to the baking sheet and toss with coconut oil and salt.

3. Sprinkle the chicken thighs generously with salt and pepper. Place the chicken thighs on top of the vegetables.

4. Bake in the oven until the chicken is cooked through, for about 30-45 minutes.

5. While the chicken is cooking, prepare the chimichurri sauce by adding all of the ingredients to a mixing bowl and whisking well.

6. Serve the roasted vegetables and chicken with chimichurri sauce.

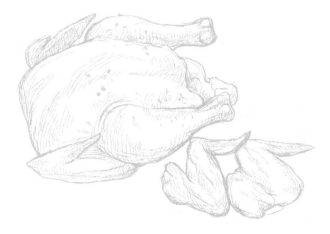

SPINACH CHICKEN

Serves: 4

Prep time: 10 minutes

Cook time: 45-50 minutes

Ingredients:

- 2 organic grass-fed chicken breast, cubed
- 3 organic grass-fed chicken thighs (skin left on, bone left in)
- 1 small yellow onion, diced
- 2 large bags fresh organic spinach
- 1 butternut squash, peeled and cut into cubes
- 1 cup organic mushrooms, chopped
- ½ cup homemade chicken stock
- 1 Tbsp. coconut oil for cooking
- Mineral salt and black pepper, freshly ground

Directions:

1. In a large pan, heat the coconut oil over medium heat. Once hot, add the onions with a pinch or two of salt to let them sweat.

2. Meanwhile, dice the chicken on a separate cutting board and season both sides with salt and pepper.

3. Add the mushrooms to the pan and let them cook for about 3-5 minutes. Then, add the spinach and cook for another 3 minutes.

4. Add the chicken, butternut squash and stock all at the same time.

5. Let this cook uncovered for 10 minutes and then cover and cook for an additional 35 minutes or until the chicken is completely cooked through.

106

OVEN-BAKED SLOPPY JOES

Serves: 4

Prep time: 10 minutes

Cook time: 3 hours

Ingredients:

- 1 lb. of organic grass-fed ground beef
- 1 small yellow onion, diced
- ¼ cup tomatoes, chopped
- 2 carrots, chopped
- ¼ cup homemade beef stock
- 1 tsp. fresh thyme, chopped
- Coconut oil for cooking
- Mineral salt and black pepper, freshly ground
- Lettuce leaves for serving

Directions:

1. Preheat the oven to 250°F.

2. Add all of the ingredients to a large roaster and gently mix.

3. Cook in the oven for 3 hours, stirring every 20 minutes.

4. Serve with lettuce leaves from the soft part of the lettuce.

GAPS MEATLOAF

Serves: 8

Prep time: 15 minutes

Cook time: 70 minutes

Tip:

- If you have any issues with nightshades, omit the tomatoes from the recipe. If you don't tolerate it, go back to previous stages.

Ingredients:

- 2 lb. organic grass-fed ground beef
- 1 organic pasture-raised egg
- ¼ cup homemade almond flour
- 1 onion, chopped
- 2 carrots, chopped
- Mineral salt and black pepper, freshly ground, to taste
- 1 Tbsp. fresh rosemary, chopped
- 1 cup tomatoes, chopped
- Coconut oil for cooking

Directions:

1. Start by preheating the oven to 350°F and greasing a loaf pan with oil. Line the pan with parchment paper to prevent sticking.

2. Add the beef and egg to a mixing bowl and mix well.

3. Add in the remaining ingredients, minus the chopped tomatoes, and mix well.

4. Place into the loaf pan and bake for about an hour.

5. While the loaf is cooking, add the chopped tomatoes to a food processor and process until smooth.

6. After one hour in the oven, remove the loaf from the oven and top it with the tomatoes. Return it to the oven for a further 10 minutes or until completely cooked through.

SIMPLE FISH TACOS

Serves: 2

Prep time: 15 minutes

Cook time: 10-15 minutes

Ingredients:

- 2 wild-caught cod fillets
- 1 avocado
- 1 small yellow onion, chopped
- 1 Tbsp. fresh cilantro, chopped
- Mineral salt and black pepper, freshly ground, to taste
- 1 Tbsp. coconut oil
- 2 large cabbage leaves

Directions:

1. Preheat the oven to 350°F and grease a baking tray with the coconut oil. Season the cod fillets with salt and pepper and place them on the baking tray. Roast for 10-15 minutes, until cooked through.

2. While the cod is cooking, add the avocado, cilantro and onion to a mixing bowl and mash.

3. Add the avocado mixture to the base of the cabbage leaves and then top with the cooked cod fillet.

4. Enjoy right away.

LEMON CHICKEN SOUP

Serves: 2-3

Prep time: 15 minutes

Cook time: 15 minutes

Ingredients:

- 2 Tbsp. grass-fed ghee
- 1 onion, chopped
- 4 cups homemade chicken stock
- 1 lb. organic pasture-raised cooked chicken thighs (Meat only, and use the meat that was cooked during the process of making homemade meatstock)
- 1 lemon, sliced
- 2 zucchinis, peeled and chopped
- 1 clove garlic, crushed
- 1 organic pasture-raised egg yolk

Directions:

1. In a large pot, warm the ghee over medium-low heat. Add the onion and salt and cook for 5 minutes, until the onions are soft but not brown.

2. Add the stock, chicken, lemon, zucchinis and garlic. Bring to a boil, then reduce the heat, cover and simmer for about 15 minutes.

3. Enjoy with an egg yolk.

ITALIAN MEATBALL STEW

Serves: 4

Prep time: 15 minutes

Cook time: 30-35 minutes

Tip:

- If you have any issues with nightshades, omit the tomatoes from the recipe.

Ingredients:

- 1 lb. organic grass-fed ground beef
- 2 Tbsp. grass-fed ghee, melted
- ¼ cup fresh parsley, chopped
- 1 tsp. Celtic sea salt
- ½ tsp. black pepper, freshly ground
- 1 lb. zucchinis, peeled and chopped
- 2 tomatoes, chopped
- ½ yellow onion, chopped
- 2 cloves garlic, chopped
- 4 cups homemade beef stock

Directions:

1. Preheat the oven to 350°F.

2. Add the zucchinis, tomatoes, onion and garlic to a large stock pot and pour the stock over the top. Bring it to a boil, then reduce the heat, cover and simmer until the vegetables are soft, for about 20 minutes.

3. Whilst the vegetables are cooking, mix the ground beef, ghee, parsley, salt and pepper together in a bowl. Form into meatballs and add to the stew once the vegetables are cooked

4. Return the stew to a boil and then simmer for a further 10 minutes.

5. Enjoy hot!

ITALIAN STUFFED ZUCCHINI BOATS

Serves: 2-3

Prep time: 10 minutes

Cook time: 20 minutes

Ingredients:

- 2 zucchinis, cut in half lengthwise
- 1 lb. organic grass-fed ground beef
- 2 cups cauliflower, finely chopped
- 1 tomato, chopped
- 1 Tbsp. lemon juice
- 2 Tbsp. fresh oregano
- ½ tsp. mineral salt
- ½ tsp. black pepper, freshly ground
- 4 cups homemade stock
- 2 Tbsp. sauerkraut

Directions:

1. Preheat the oven to 350°F.

2. In a large pot, add the beef, cauliflower, tomato, stock, lemon juice, oregano, salt and pepper.

3. Bring the stock to a boil, cover and then simmer for 20 minutes or until the beef and vegetables are cooked through.

4. Scoop out the inside of the zucchinis and place them in a 9 x 9 casserole dish.

5. Bake the zucchinis in the oven for 25-30 minutes or until the zucchinis are tender.

6. Using a slotted spoon, scoop the beef mixture out of the stock and divide it between the zucchini boats.

7. Serve immediately, while the zucchini boats and beef mixture are both still hot.

Tip:

- If you have any issues with nightshades, omit the tomatoes from the recipe. Cooked and peeled beetroot may be used instead of tomatoes.

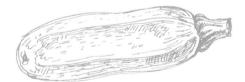

ROASTED CHICKEN AND EGGPLANT WITH HERB SAUCE

Serves: 4

Prep time: 10 minutes

Cook time: 30-40 minutes

Ingredients:

- 1 lb. organic pasture-raised chicken thighs
- 1 eggplant, peeled and cut into bite-sized cubes
- 2 cups grape or cherry tomatoes
- 3 Tbsp. coconut oil, melted
- 1 tsp. dried oregano
- ¾ tsp. mineral salt
- 1 cup homemade fish stock
- ½ onion, chopped
- ½ cup fresh parsley, chopped
- 2 Tbsp. lemon juice

Directions:

1. Preheat the oven to 350°F. Line a standard baking sheet with parchment paper.

2. Place the chicken thighs on half of the baking sheet and the eggplant and tomatoes on the other half. Drizzle the chicken and vegetables with the coconut oil, oregano and a quarter teaspoon of salt.

3. Bake for 30-40 minutes, or until chicken and eggplant are cooked through.

4. To make the sauce, bring the fish stock to a simmer in a large skillet. Add the onion, cover and cook for 5-10 minutes or until the onion is softened.

5. Add the cooked onion and stock to a blender with the parsley, lemon juice and the remaining half teaspoon of salt. Blend until smooth. Add more fish stock if the sauce is not blending well.

6. Serve the chicken, eggplant and tomatoes topped with the sauce.

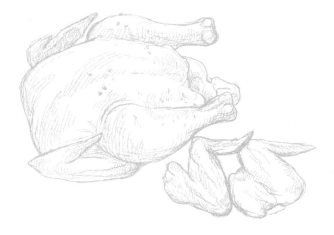

SNACKS

CINNAMON APPLESAUCE

Serves: 4

Prep time: 15 minutes

Cook time: 20-25 minutes

Ingredients:

- 4 ripe apples, peeled and cored
- 3 Tbsp. grass-fed ghee
- ½ tsp. ground cinnamon
- ¼ cup filtered water

Directions:

1. Start by peeling and coring the apples and add them to a stockpot with the filtered water until soft. This should take 20-25 minutes.

2. Once the apples are soft, add the ghee and cinnamon to the stockpot and mash with a potato masher.

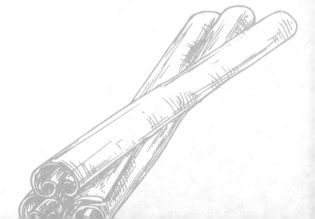

MINT PINEAPPLE MANGO JUICE

Serves: 2

Prep time: 5 minutes

Cook time: 0 minutes

Tip:

- If you do not have a juicer, you can make juice in a high-speed blender and then strain it using a fine mesh strainer after blending.

Ingredients:

- 2 ripe mangoes, sliced
- 1 cup fresh pineapple, cubed
- 1 handful fresh mint leaves

Directions:

1. Run all of the ingredients through a juicer.

2. If the juice contains clumps, you can run the juice through a fine mesh strainer before dividing it between two glasses.

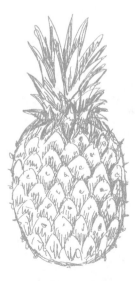

APPLE CELERY JUICE

Serves: 2

Prep time: 5 minutes

Cook time: 0 minutes

Tip:

- If you do not have a juicer, you can make juice in a high-speed blender and then strain it using a fine mesh strainer after blending.

Ingredients:

- 3 ripe apples, peeled and cored
- 4 stalks celery

Directions:

1. Run the apples and celery stalks through a juicer.

2. If the juice contains clumps, you can run the juice through a fine mesh strainer.

3. Divide it between two glasses.

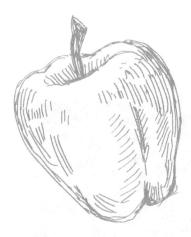

SEA SALT BAKED KALE CHIPS

Serves: 6

Prep time: 15 minutes

Cook time: 30-40 minutes

Ingredients:

- 1 bunch kale, washed and stems removed
- 2 Tbsp. coconut oil, melted
- 1 tsp. mineral salt

Directions:

1. Start by preheating the oven to 250°F and lining a baking sheet with parchment paper.

2. Remove the stems from the kale leaves and then wash and pat dry.

3. Rip the kale leaves into small pieces and evenly distribute them onto the baking sheet.

4. Drizzle the kale leaves with the melted coconut oil and season with the sea salt.

5. Bake for 30-40 minutes or until the kale chips are crispy.

Stage 6

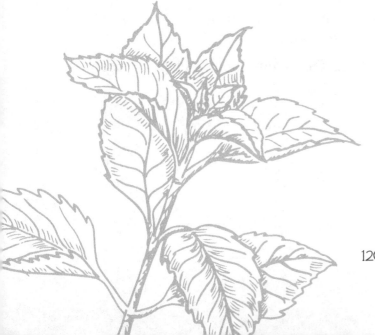

BREAKFAST

MINTY GREEN SMOOTHIE

Serves: 1

Prep time: 5 minutes

Cook time: 0 minutes

Ingredients:

- ½ avocado
- 2 cups fresh spinach
- 1 cup full-fat unsweetened coconut milk (homemade or purchased in a glass jar with no preservatives)
- ¼ cup fresh mint leaves
- 1-inch piece fresh ginger, peeled
- Juice from ½ lime

Directions:

1. Add all ingredients into a high-speed blender and blend until smooth. If the smoothie is too thick, add more coconut milk or water.

2. Pour into a glass and enjoy straight away.

BANANA PUMPKIN SMOOTHIE

Serves: 1

Prep time: 5 minutes

Cook time: 0 minutes

Ingredients:

- 1 ripe banana with brown spots on the skin
- 1 cup full-fat unsweetened coconut milk (homemade or purchased in a glass jar with no preservatives)
- ¼ cup cooked pumpkin (steamed or roasted)
- 2 pitted dates

Directions:

1. Add all ingredients into a high-speed blender and blend until smooth. If the smoothie is too thick, add more coconut milk or water.

2. Pour into a glass and enjoy straight away.

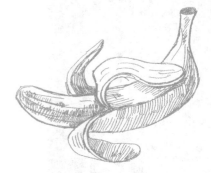

ROASTED SQUASH FRITTATA MUFFINS

Serves: 12

Prep time: 10 minutes

Cook time: 35-40 minutes

Ingredients:

- 9 organic pasture-raised eggs
- 1 tsp. dried oregano
- ¼ tsp. mineral salt
- ½ cup kale, chopped
- ½ cup fresh parsley, chopped
- 1 cup winter squash, roasted and cubed

Directions:

1. Start by preheating the oven to 325°F and lining a standard muffin tin with muffin cups or greasing it with coconut oil.

2. In a large bowl, whisk together the eggs, oregano and salt. Mix in the parsley, kale and squash.

3. Divide the egg mixture into the muffin tin. Bake for 35-40 minutes or until the eggs have set.

4. Enjoy with a side of avocado and homemade stock.

CINNAMON ALMOND FLOUR MUFFINS

Serves: 12

Prep time: 10 minutes

Cook time: 15-20 minutes

Ingredients:

- 2 ½ cups homemade almond flour
- 3 organic pasture-raised eggs
- ¼ cup unsweetened homemade apple sauce
- 2 Tbsp. raw honey
- 2 Tbsp. coconut oil, melted
- 1 tsp. ground cinnamon
- ½ cup dried fruit of choice (no sugar or additives)

Directions:

1. Start by preheating the oven to 350°F and lining a standard muffin tin with muffin cups or greasing it with coconut oil.

2. In a large bowl, whisk together the dry ingredients and then fold in the eggs, apple sauce, coconut oil and raw honey. Stir well.

3. Pour the batter into the muffin tins and bake for 15-20 minutes or until a toothpick inserted into the center comes out clean.

4. Allow to cool and enjoy as an easy breakfast.

LUNCH

CARROT GINGER SOUP

Serves: 6

Prep time: 10 minutes

Cook time: 30-35 minutes

Ingredients:

- 2 Tbsp. coconut oil
- 2 yellow onions, chopped
- 1 apple, peeled and grated
- 1 ½ lbs. carrots, chopped
- ½ tsp. mineral salt
- 4 cups homemade stock
- 2 Tbsp. lemon juice, freshly squeezed
- 1 Tbsp. fresh ginger, grated

Directions:

1. In a large pot over medium heat, add the coconut oil. Add in the onion, carrots, apple and salt and cook until they soften, for about 8 minutes.

2. Add the stock and bring to a boil, then reduce the heat to low and simmer for 25 minutes or until the carrots are tender.

3. Use an immersion stick or a blender and blend until smooth. Stir in the lemon juice and ginger.

4. Taste and add more salt, if needed

EGG SALAD STUFFED PEPPER

Serves: 2

Prep time: 15 minutes

Cook time: 0 minutes

Ingredients:

- 1 red bell pepper
- 1 avocado, pitted and peeled
- 4 organic pasture-raised eggs, soft-boiled
- 1 small apple, cored and chopped
- ¼ cup fresh parsley, chopped
- 2 Tbsp. lemon or lime juice
- ¼ tsp. mineral salt

Directions:

1. Remove the stem and cut the red bell pepper in half lengthwise. Remove the seeds and set aside.

2. In a medium bowl, add the eggs and avocado and mash with a fork. Mix in the apple, parsley, lemon or lime juice and salt.

3. Taste and add more salt or lemon/lime juice, if needed.

4. Scoop the salad into the red bell pepper halves and enjoy with a warm glass of homemade stock!

LAMB MEATBALLS

Serves: 8

Prep time: 15 minutes

Cook time: 20 minutes

Ingredients:

- 1 lb. organic grass-fed ground lamb
- 1 organic pasture-raised egg
- ½ tsp. ground cumin
- ½ tsp. ground cinnamon
- ¼ tsp. allspice
- 1 tsp. mineral salt
- 6 Roma tomatoes, diced
- ¼ cup coconut oil for cooking
- Fresh cilantro for serving

Directions:

1. Start by preheating the oven to 350°F and lining a baking sheet with parchment paper.

2. Add all of the ingredients, minus the tomatoes, olive oil and cilantro, to a large mixing bowl and mix well.

3. Place the meatballs onto the parchment lined baking sheet and bake for about 20 minutes or until cooked through, flipping halfway through.

4. While the meatballs are cooking, chop the tomatoes and add to a stockpot with the coconut oil. Simmer for about 10 minutes or until the tomatoes are tender.

5. Once the meatballs are cooked, serve with the tomatoes and fresh cilantro.

Tip:

- If you have any issues with nightshades, omit the tomatoes from the recipe and go back in stages to support additional healing. Cooked and peeled beetroot may be used instead of tomatoes.

ROSEMARY CHICKEN APPLE SALAD

Serves: 2

Prep time: 15 minutes

Cook time: 0 minutes

Tip:

- Leave the yogurt out if dairy is not tolerated.

Ingredients:

- 2 cups organic pasture-raised chicken, cooked and shredded
- 1 green apple, peeled, cored and roughly chopped
- 2 tsp. dried rosemary
- 2 Tbsp. olive oil
- 1 Tbsp. homemade yogurt (if tolerated)
- 1 Tbsp. lemon juice
- ½ tsp. mineral salt
- 2 cups lettuce, chopped

Directions:

1. In a medium bowl, add the chicken, apple, rosemary, olive oil, yogurt (if using), lemon juice and salt. Mix until thoroughly combined.

2. Serve on top of a bed of lettuce.

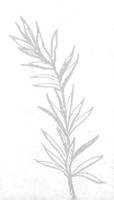

DINNER

COCONUT CHICKEN

Serves: 4

Prep time: 15 minutes +
chilling time (1-4 hours)

Cook time: 30-40 minutes

Ingredients:

- 6 organic grass-fed chicken thighs (skin left on, bone left in)
- 2 organic grass-fed chicken breasts, cubed
- 1/2 cup organic full-fat coconut milk (homemade or purchased in a glass jar with no preservatives)
- 1 Tbsp. turmeric powder
- 1 Tbsp. ground cumin
- 1 clove garlic, peeled
- 1 small yellow onion, chopped
- 4 Tbsp. coconut oil for marinade
- 2 Tbsp. grass-fed ghee for cooking
- Mineral salt and black pepper, freshly ground
- Fresh cilantro for serving, if desired.

Directions:

1. In a food processor add the spices, garlic, coconut milk, coconut oil, salt and pepper. Blend until the desired consistency is reached, about 80% smooth. Add the marinade to a resealable container.

2. Season the chicken lightly with sea salt and add it to the marinade in the container before placing it in the refrigerator for at least an hour - 4 hours is recommended.

3. Once you have marinated the chicken, remove it from the refrigerator while you prepare the other items.

4. Finely chop the onion. Add the ghee to a large saucepan over medium heat and then, once the ghee has melted, add the onions with a pinch of salt.

5. Once the onions are translucent, turn off the heat. Add the chicken and half of the marinade from the container.

6. Arrange the chicken and onion mixture on a parchment-lined baking sheet, spacing out the chicken.

7. Preheat the oven to 375 degrees F and bake for 30-40 minutes or until completely cooked through.

8. Halfway through the cooking time, turn each piece over and add the rest of the marinade from the container.

9. Once the chicken is completely cooked, remove it from the oven.

10. Garnish with fresh cilantro, if desired.

"SPAGHETTI" AND MEATBALLS

Serves: 4

Prep time: 15 minutes

Cook time: 45 minutes

Tip:

- If you have any issues with nightshades, this recipe may be best avoided due to the diced tomatoes included in the recipe. If not tolerated, go back in stages.

Ingredients:

- 4 zucchinis, peeled, and spiralized
- 1 organic pasture-raised egg
- ¼ cup homemade almond flour
- 3 cloves garlic, minced
- 1 tsp. dried oregano
- ½ tsp. fennel seeds
- ½ tsp. mineral salt
- 1 lb. organic grass-fed ground beef
- 2 Tbsp. coconut oil, melted
- 28 ounces of diced tomatoes
- ½ cup homemade beef stock

Directions:

1. Start by adding the diced tomatoes, spiralized zucchini, and stock to a pan and simmer until the sauce thickens, for about 30 minutes.

2. While the ssauce is cooking, whisk the egg, almond flour, garlic, oregano, fennel and salt together in a large bowl.

3. Add the ground beef and use your hands to thoroughly combine. Roll into 1.5 inch meatballs.

4. Place the meatballs on a parchment-lined baking sheet about 1 inch apart and bake at 375 degrees F for 20 minutes or until they are cooked through.

TURKEY AND EGGPLANT BOLOGNESE

Serves: 4

Prep time: 15 minutes

Cook time: 90 minutes

Tip:
- If you have any issues with nightshades, this recipe may be best avoided due to the tomato sauce included in the recipe. If not tolerated, go back in stages.

Ingredients:

- 1 lb. organic grass-fed ground turkey
- 1 small yellow onion, diced
- 2 small organic carrots, diced
- 2/3 -3/4 cup organic eggplant, peeled and diced
- 1-2 large cloves garlic, minced
- ½ cup organic red bell pepper, diced
- 2 cups organic (no preservative) tomato sauce from a glass jar only
- 3 Tbsp. grass-fed ghee
- Mineral salt and black pepper, freshly ground, to taste

Directions:

1. Preheat the oven to 400°F. Add the tomato sauce and ghee to a casserole dish with a heavy lid

2. Use your hands to break up with turkey mince as you add it to the casserole dish. Stir the meat into the sauce until well covered. Add the rest of the ingredients to the casserole dish and stir again.

3. Fold a sheet of aluminum foil in half and place it under the lid before pressing the lid down over the casserole dish. The foil should create a seal.

4. Cook in the oven for 1½ hours, until a thick and rich sauce is formed.

CUBAN BEEF

Serves: 3

Prep time: 15 minutes

Cook time: 20-25 minutes

Ingredients:

- 3/4 lb. organic grass-fed beef, cubed and stewed
- 1 small yellow onion, diced
- 1 green bell pepper, diced
- 2 cloves garlic, minced
- 1 tsp. dried oregano
- Mineral salt and black pepper, freshly ground, to taste
- Coconut oi for cooking

Directions:

1. Add the coconut oil to a skillet over medium heat. Once hot, add the onion with 2 pinches of sea salt to let them sweat.

2. Add the green bell pepper and garlic to the sauté pan. Season with salt and pepper and cook for 5-7 minutes, ensuring that there is enough olive oil to avoid the vegetables burning.

3. Season the beef with salt and pepper and place the beef under a medium grill. Cook the beef according to preference.

4. Mix the beef and the vegetables together and serve hot.

CHICKEN BREAST WITH SUMMER SQUASH

Serves: 4

Prep time: 15 minutes

Cook time: 25-30 minutes

Ingredients:

- 4 organic grass-fed chicken breasts
- 1 large lemon, sliced
- 2 Tbsp. capers, rinsed and drained
- 2 cups organic yellow squash, peeled and diced
- 8- 10 organic zucchinis, peeled and diced
- 1 cup organic asparagus, quartered
- 1/3 cup flat leaf organic parsley, chopped
- 6 Tbsp. coconut oil, melted
- Mineral salt and black pepper, freshly ground, to taste

Directions:

1. Preheat the oven to 350°F. Line a baking sheet with parchment paper.

2. Place the chicken breasts on the baking sheet, season with salt, pepper and half the coconut oil.

3. Garnish with slices of lemon and capers.

4. Bake in the oven for 25-30 minutes or until cooked through.

5. While the chicken is cooking, add the remaining coconut oil to a skillet over medium heat and carefully add the vegetables. Season with salt and pepper and cook until the vegetables are tender, for about 6-7 minutes.

6. Turn the heat off, add the parsley and gently toss.

7. Serve the baked chicken with a squeeze of lemon and the vegetables.

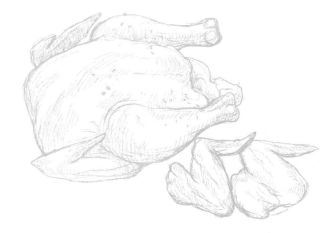

SNACKS

TRAIL MIX

Serves: 8

Prep time: 10 minutes

Cook time: 0 minutes

Ingredients:

- 1 cup of unsalted organic pumpkin seeds
- 1 cup of raw almonds
- ½ cup organic raisins
- 3 Tbsp. raw honey
- 1 tsp. mineral salt

Directions:

1. Add all the ingredients minus the raw honey and salt to a large mixing bowl and toss to combine.

2. Add the salt and raw honey and mix.

3. Enjoy and store leftovers in a mason-style jar.

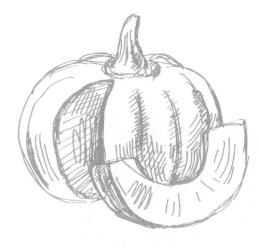

BERRIES AND COCONUT CREAM

Serves: 1

Prep time: 5 minutes

Cook time: 0 minutes

Ingredients:

- ¼ cup full-fat coconut cream (homemade or store bough in a glass jar only with no preservatives)
- ¼ cup mixed berries
- 1 tsp. raw honey

Directions:

1. Simply add the coconut cream to a bowl and top with the mixed berries.

2. Drizzle with raw honey and enjoy.

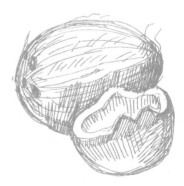

BAKED CINNAMON APPLE

Serves: 2

Prep time: 10 minutes

Cook time: 25-30 minutes

Ingredients:

- 4 apples, cored and peeled
- ½ tsp. ground cinnamon
- ½ Tbsp. raw honey
- ½ Tbsp. grass-fed ghee
- ½ cup walnuts, crushed
- 1 cup filtered water

Directions:

1. Preheat the oven to 350°F.

2. Add all of the ingredients, minus the apples, to a small bowl and mix well.

3. Stuff the core of each apple with a quarter of the sweet filling.

4. Place the apples in a deep baking dish, add the water and place the dish in the oven.

5. Bake for 25-30 minutes and serve warm with some homemade sour cream.

YOGURT MANGO PARFAIT

Serves: 1

Prep time: 5 minutes

Cook time: 0 minutes

Ingredients:

- ½ cup of homemade yogurt
- 1 ripe mango, cubed
- 1 tsp. raw honey

Directions:

1. Start by adding the yogurt to a bowl and top with the cubed mango.

2. Drizzle with raw honey and enjoy.

COOKING CONVERSION TABLES

Spoon, Cups	Liquid - ml
1/4 tsp.	1.25 ml
1/2 tsp.	2.5 ml
1 tsp.	5 ml
1 Tbsp.	15 ml
1/4 cup	60 ml
1/3 cup	80 ml
1/2 cup	125 ml
1 cup	250 ml

Dry Measurements		
1 Tbsp.	1/2 ounce	14g
1/4 cup	2 ounce	56.7g
1/3 cup	2.6 ounce	75.4g
1/2 cup	4 ounces	113.4
3/4 cup	6 ounces	170g
1 cup	8 ounces	227g
2 cups	16 ounces	454g

Volume Liquid		
2 Tbsp.	1 fl. oz.	30 ml
1/4 cup	2 fl. oz.	60 ml
1/2 cup	4 fl. oz.	125 ml
1 cup	8 fl. oz.	250 ml
1.5 cups	12 fl. oz.	375 ml
2 cups/1 pint	16 fl. oz.	500 ml
4 cups/1 quart	32 fl. oz.	1000 ml / 1 litre

Made in United States
North Haven, CT
29 June 2024